SEX, PERFORMANCE, REPRODUCTION, NAKED RADICALS AND ANTIOXIDANTS

A SELECTIVE REVIEW

BY
PROF. HON. RANDOLPH M. HOWES, M.D., Ph.D.

Physician, Surgeon and Scientist (Biochemist)

Adjunct Assistant Professor of Plastic Surgery,
The Johns Hopkins Hospital, Baltimore, MD USA

Espaldon Professor of Plastic and Reconstructive Surgery,
University of Santo Tomas, Manila, Philippines

Adjunct Professor of Biological Sciences,
Southeastern Louisiana University

Vice Chancellor/Dean, Louisiana University of Medical Sciences
(Also holds an Honorary Doctorate of Humanities, SLU)

DOC
R ANDOLPH
 x
HOWES

RAD!CAL

NOTICE TO USERS:

It is understood that medicine is an ever-changing science. As new research and clinical experience broaden our knowledge, changes in treatment and drug therapy are required. The author and the publisher of this work have checked with sources believed to be reliable in their efforts to provide information that is complete and generally in accord with the standards accepted at the time of publication. However, in view of the possibility of human error or changes in the medical sciences, neither the authors nor the publisher nor any other party who has been involved in the preparation of publication of this work warrants that the information contained herein is in every respect accurate or complete, and they disclaim all responsibility to any errors or omissions or for the results obtained from use of the information contained in the work. Readers should confirm the information contained herein with other sources. For example and in particular, readers are advised to check the product information sheets (or labels) included in the package of each drug they plan to administer to be certain that the information contained in this work is accurate and that changes have not been made in the recommended dose or in the contraindications for administration. This recommendation is of particular importance in connection with new or infrequently used drugs, additives or supplements.

DISCLAIMERS:

Please note: only your personal physician or other health professional you consult can best advise you on matters of your health based on your medical history, your family medical history, your medication history, and how information from any of these databases may apply to you. Neither Dr. Howes nor any party involved in creating, producing or delivering this web site shall be liable for any damages arising out of access to or use of this material or web site, or any errors or omissions in the content thereof.

FINANCIAL DISCLOSURE:

Dr. Howes has no financial conflicts of interest and is not involved in the sale of dietary supplements or fitness equipment. The author holds no stocks or interests in companies in the food additive or antioxidant supplement business.

The story of antioxidants,
as they relate to disease
prevention, cure, and antiaging
is the story of ….
FAILURE!

R. M. Howes, M.D., Ph.D.
6/2/11

ABOUT THE AUTHOR
Dr. Randolph M. Howes M.D., Ph.D.

BIOGRAPHICAL SKETCH:

As a champion of the people, Dr. Howes anticipates and hopes for the active involvement of all connected parties (patients, caregivers, healthcare professionals, etc.) as an integral approach to educating consumers and the public about the potential dangers of excessive antioxidant-containing supplements and "antioxidant stacking."

Some people are born with a silver spoon in their mouth but Dr. Howes had to earn his. Even as a child, Dr. Howes could think with adult clarity. He could envision his future but it would require "decades of dedication" to make it a reality.

From childhood, Dr. Howes was motivated to become a medical doctor and scientist. Assuredly, having been born on a small strawberry farm in rural Louisiana, his journey to the top has proved to be arduous and demanding.

However, he was fortunate to acquire the confidence of Sister Elizabeth at St. Joseph's school and went on to gain the support of his high school speech teacher, Mrs. Iris Brann, who also had strong beliefs in his abilities and potential. Ultimately, with the help of his guitar and his singing ability, he defeated the star quarter back of the high school football team to become the president of the student body.

With the aid of a $25 dollar legislative scholarship, he went on to Southeastern Louisiana College (SLC). At SLC, he was selected for honors chemistry, made the Dean's list, worked at the Psychology Research Lab forty hours a week, maintained a premed study load, and was elected president of the Junior Class and the Interfraternity Council.

To earn badly needed funds, he played music on weekends in a small combo, The Three Blind Mice. Next, he matriculated to Tulane University School of Medicine.

His initial dream was to try to combine both medicine and science. In that regard, he began work as a technician with Dr. Andrew Schally at the Endocrine Polypeptide Lab in the isolation of thyrotropin releasing factor. This work led to a Nobel Prize for Dr. Schally.

Dr. Howes had been highly impressed with the enthusiasm of biochemist, Dr. Richard H. Steele, who accepted him as a doctoral candidate under his tutelage. Dr. Howes graduated in the top 10 of his class, won the Louisiana Pathology Association Award, was elected to the Sigma Xi honor fraternity and was the first in the history of Tulane to become a Doctor of Medicine and a Ph.D. in biochemistry concurrently.

Next, he was selected to pursue a career in surgery at the prestigious Johns Hopkins Hospital.

Unbelievably, at Dr. Howes' urging, he was allowed to operate his own research lab during his surgical internship and residency training while at Johns Hopkins Hospital. He worked hand in hand with the greats in American medicine and surgery.

Independently, he garnered grants, trained lab techs, wrote papers, slept on the cold floor, proudly served as a Captain in the U.S. Army Reserves Medical Corp and finished with board eligibility in both general and plastic surgery in an unheard of six year period.

In another first, he was appointed as an Adjunct Assistant Professor of Plastic Surgery at Johns Hopkins Hospital.

For decades, Dr. Howes gave unselfishly to pro bono medical missions in the Philippines and he holds the Ernesto Espaldon Chair as Professor of Plastic Surgery at the University of Santo Tomas.

Upon retirement from a career in cosmetic plastic surgery, he is living his dream of trying to revolutionize the treatment of cancer, heart disease, HIV/

AIDS and malaria, with his in depth knowledge of the arcane biochemistry of oxygen metabolism. He is a work in progress! Dedicated and passionate, he is on a mission for mankind.

Dr. Howes invented the triple lumen venous catheter, which has been credited with helping save the lives of over 20 million critically ill patients worldwide. His catheter became the number one venous catheter in the world and his name is well recognized in over 100 countries. He has been recognized as a humanitarian, visionary, entrepreneur, singer, songwriter, inventor and author.

He received the Harper Award for innovative research from the American College for Advancement in Medicine, served as their keynote speaker and his peers refer to him as "a walking encyclopedia on oxygen metabolism."

He is a Dr. Norman Vincent Peale Unsung Hero award winner, which recognized his awesome versatility. Additionally, even though he is humble and does not like talking about it, he is a self made multi-millionaire.

He is currently doing extensive research on cures for cancer and heart disease and development of revolutionary treatment modalities. He has written 16 books over the past 8 years on the subject of oxygen metabolism, as it relates to protection from cancer, heart disease, diabetes, malaria, HIV/AIDS, Alzheimer's disease, aging and arthritis. He has written many scientific and medical papers and has lectured nationally and internationally.

His research has shown that currently common antioxidant vitamins, such as vitamins A & E, (and vitamin C to a lesser extent) can be harmful and that oxygen free radicals protect us from bacterial, fungal and viral infections and they help to control cancer growth.

He has developed an effective, inexpensive singlet oxygen generating system, from orthomolecular agents, for the treatment of cancer and heart disease. He is passionate about his research and hopes to have his discoveries at the patient's bedside in his lifetime. Admittedly, this is an extremely ambitious goal.

There are over 10,000 pages in his magnum opus and at the Howes World Selective Library on Oxygen Metabolism. **Over 3,000 pages of his opus are available online in a searchable format www.iwillfindthecure.org** © by R.M. Howes

NOTE: An avid researcher, Dr. Howes has authored more than 300 original publications, including about 30 medical and scientific books, such as Death In Small Doses (Antioxidant vitamins A, C & E in the 21st Century), Antioxidant Overkill and Dangers of Excessive Antioxidants In Cancer Patients. He has written numerous articles for medical and consumer publications, including The Journal of American Academy of Cosmetic Surgery, Annals of the New York Academy of Science, The Journal of Evidence Based Complementary And Alternative Medicine, The Baton Rouge Advocate, and The Houma Courier. He has a weekly science/medicine column in the Hammond Daily Star and The Ponchatoula Times. His research interests include truthful reporting of antioxidant dangers, adverse effects of vitamins A, C & E, other antioxidant's deadly unintended consequences, free radicals, oxygen metabolism, and cancer and heart disease treatment and prevention, global health care policy, and oxidative means to revolutionize treating and preventing HIV/AIDS and malaria.

Dr. Howes is also an active and well-known speaker and media personality, having been featured on PBS's The American Health Journal, WWL-TV New Orleans and WDSU-TV New Orleans, Sirius/XM satellite radio, as well as many other national talk and news shows across America.

The scientific method demands that we change our beliefs or theories to fit the factual data. I believe that this applies directly to the Free Radi-Crap theory. Again, I say to you, "The free radical theory has fallen and so has the mitochondrial free radical theory of aging."

COMPANION PAPERS:

Citation: R. M. Howes: Mythology of Antioxidant Vitamins?. *The Journal of Evidence-Based Alternative and Complimentary Medicine.* April, 2011. 16(2): 149-189.

Citation: R. M. Howes: Cancer Therapy: A Review with Scientific Validation for the Role of Electronically Modified Oxygen Derivatives in Oncologic Treatment Modalities. *The Internet Journal of Alternative Medicine.* 2010 Volume 8 Number I.

Citation: R. M. Howes: Hydrogen Peroxide: A review of a scientifically verifiable omnipresent ubiquitous essentiality of obligate, aerobic, carbon-based life forms. *The Internet Journal of Plastic Surgery.* 2010 Volume 7 Number I.

Howes M.D., PhD., R. (2009). Dangers of Antioxidants in Cancer Patients: A Review. *PHILICA.COM Article number 153.* Published 7th February, 2009. (20 pages)

Howes M.D., PhD., R. (2008). Aging and anti-aging claims: a review on antioxidant vitamins A, C & E. *PHILICA.COM Article number 116.* Published on 12th January, 2008. (16 pages)

Howes M.D., PhD., R. (2007). Sleep: An original "radical" proposal. *PHILICA.COM Observation number 42.* Published on 5th October, 2007. (1 page)

Howes M.D., PhD., R. (2007). Antioxidant Vitamins A, C & E; Death in Small Doses and Legal Liability? *PHILICA.COM Article number 89.* Published on 5th April, 2007. (23 pages)

Howes M.D., PhD., R. (2007). Cancer, Apoptosis and Reactive Oxygen Species: A New Paradigm. *PHILICA.COM Article number 86.* Published on 26th February, 2007. (11 pages)

Howes M.D., PhD., R. (2007). Antioxidant Vitamins A, C and E: Assessing Potential for Harm. *PHILICA.COM Article number 83.* Published on 15th February, 2007. (14 pages)

Howes M.D., PhD., R. (2007). The Consequent Downfall of the Free Radical Theory. *PHILICA.COM Article number 75*. Published on 22nd January, 2007. (9 pages)

Howes, R.M.: "The Free Radical Fantasy," The Annals of New York Academy of Sciences, 2006, Vol. 1067, pp. 22-26.

OTHER BOOKS PUBLISHED:
Partial list

The Fire Eaters, Molding your own destiny more easily, Carnivore Press, © 1982

Uplift, The Answer Book to your plastic and cosmetic surgery questions, Carnivore Press, © 1986

The Pundit Speaks, Vol. I. An Anthology of Neoclassical Poetic Philosophy, Carnivore Press, © 1990

The Pundit Speaks, Volume II, An Anthology of Neoclassical Poetic Philosophy, Free Radical Press, © 1994

The Pundit Speaks, Volume III, An Anthology of Neoclassical Poetic Philosophy, Free Radical Press, © 1996

The Fable of the Chocolate Covered Strawberry Coloring Book Free Radical Press, © 2001

The Pundit Speaks, Volume IV, An Anthology of Neoclassical Poetic Philosophy, Free Radical Press, © 2003

U.T.O.P.I.A. Unified Theory of Oxygen Participation In Aerobiosis Free Radical Publishing Co, © 2004 (e-book) 767 pages

The Medical and Scientific Significance of Oxygen Free Radical Metabolism, Free Radical Publishing Co, © 2005 (e-book) 934 pages

Hydrogen Peroxide: Monograph I: Scientific, Medical & Biochemical Overview & Antioxidant Vitamins A, C & E 200 pages Monograph 2: Equivocal Scientific Studies, Free Radical Publishing Co, © 2006 (e-book) 171 pages

Cardiovascular Disease & Oxygen Free Radical Mythology, Free Radical Publishing Co, © 2006 (e-book) 308 pages

Diabetes and Oxygen Free Radical Sophistry, Free Radical Publishing Co, © 2006 (e-book) 366 pages

Reactive Oxygen Species Insufficiency (ROSI) as the Basis for Coexistent Diseases: Extraordinary Support for an Extraordinary Theory. Volume I - 501 pages Volume II, - 505 pages Volume III, Free Radical Publishing Co, © 2008 (e-books) 562 pages ~ 1564 pages total

Coffee Table Musings Of The Da Vinci in Cowboy Boots. Pithy Prose and Perspicacious Aphorisms. Trafford Publishing, © 2009 (108 pages)

THE HOWES PAPERS. Free Radical Publishing Co, © 2009 (e-book) 211 pages

The Pundit Speaks, Volume V, An Anthology of Neoclassical Poetic Philosophy, Trafford Publishing, © 2010 (164 pages)

Death in Small Doses? Antioxidant Vitamins A, C and E in the Twenty-first Century: A Heath Impact Statement for the Layman. Book One, Trafford Publishing, © 2010 (348 pages for Books 1 and 2 combined)

Death in Small Doses? Antioxidant Vitamins A, C and E are Making a Killing. A Health Impact Statement for the Medical Scientist. Book Two, Trafford Publishing, © 2010

Reactive Oxygen Species vs. Antioxidants: "The Oxypocalypse" or "The war that never was." Free Radical Publishing Co, © 2010 (e-book) 550 pages

Antioxidant Vitamins: Vitamins A, C & E - Negligible Results, Half Truths and Potential Harm as Demonstrated by Failed Intervention Trials. Free Radical Publishing Co, © 2010 (e-book) 236 pages

Radically Change Your Thinking About Oxygen. Free Radical Publishing Co, © 2010 (e-book) 366 pages

EMODS: The New Radical Strategy. Free Radical Publishing Co, © 2010 (e-book) 300 pages

Antioxidant Overkill: An antioxidant guide for the educated consumer. CreateSpace and Free Radical Publishing Co. USA, © 2011 (428 pages)

Dangers of Excessive Antioxidants In Cancer Patients. CreateSpace and Free Radical Publishing Co, USA, © 2011 (512 pages)

Heart Disease and Antioxidant Failures. CreateSpace and Free Radical Publishing Co, USA, © 2011 (634 pages)

Antioxidant Failures and Dangers: The Consequent Fall of the Free Radical Theory. CreateSpace and Free Radical Publishing Co, USA, © 2011 (434 pages)

Anti-aging Anti-oxidant Scams: A Radical Scheme. CreateSpace and Free Radical Publishing Co, USA, © 2011 (332 pages)

Sports, Athletes, Exercise Facts and Antioxidant Myths. CreateSpace and Free Radical Publishing Co, USA © 2011(422 pages)

Alzheimer's Disease: Forget Antioxidants and Supplements. CreateSpace and Free Radical Publishing Co, USA, © 2012 (362 pages)

Antioxidant Links To Deadly Unintended Consequences. CreateSpace and Free Radical Publishing Co, USA, © 2012 (341 pages)

The Nth Degree. A Novel, Sci-Fi Series, #1 Parallel Universe Series, CreateSpace and Free Radical Publishing Co, USA © 2012 (230 pages)

Slightly Green. A Novel, Sci-Fi Series, #2 Parallel Universe Series, CreateSpace and Free Radical Publishing Co, USA, © 2012 (200 pages)

Ultiminium. A Novel, Sci-Fi Series, #3 Parallel Universe Series, CreateSpace and Free Radical Publishing Co, USA, © 2012 (200 pages)

The Believer's Question: That God Thingy. A Novel, Sci-Fi Series, #4 Parallel Universe Series, CreateSpace and Free Radical Publishing Co, USA, © 2012

Pangaea 6. A Novel, Sci-Fi Series, #5 Parallel Universe Series CreateSpace and Free Radical Publishing Co, USA, © 2012 (174 pages)

Catching Cancer. A Novel, Sci-Fi Series, #6 Parallel Universe Series, CreateSpace and Free Radical Publishing Co, USA, © 2012 (140 pages)

Tulane Voodoo. A Novel, Sci-Fi Series, #7 Parallel Universe Series, CreateSpace and Free Radical Publishing Co, USA, © 2012 (144 pages)

The Saints' Curse and Ghosts on the Levee. A Novel, Sci-Fi Series, #8 Parallel Universe Series, CreateSpace and Free Radical Publishing Co, USA, © 2012

LSU Spirit, in the Mounds. A Novel, Sci-Fi Series,#9 Parallel Universe Series, CreateSpace and Free Radical Publishing Co, USA, © 2012 (152 pages)

AVAILABLE AT:

www.philica.com
www.medi.philica.com
www.iwillfindthecure.org
www.amazon.com
www.BarnesandNobles.com

DEDICATION

To life's incredible journey....a journey of discovery!

Dr. Mehmet OoZe presents his daily, hour-long, TV infomercial, "Hawking The Supplements"

R.M. Howes M.D., Ph.D.
3/3/12

TABLE OF CONTENTS

CHAPTER THREE

CHAPTER FOUR

CHAPTER FIVE

CHAPTER SIX

CHAPTER SEVEN

CHAPTER EIGHT

CHAPTER NINE

CHAPTER TEN

CHAPTER ELEVEN

CHAPTER TWELVE

CHAPTER THIRTEEN

CHAPTER FOURTEEN

CHAPTER FIFTEEN

CHAPTER SIXTEEN

CHAPTER SEVENTEEN

CHAPTER EIGHTTEEN

CHAPTER NINTEEN

CHAPTER TWENTY

CHAPTER TWENTY ONE

CHAPTER TWENTY TWO

CHAPTER TWENTY THREE

CHAPTER ONE

The most important and the largest sex organ is located between the ears…..and is commonly referred to as "the brain." Libido is a function of testosterone and erection is a function of free radicals.

An overall view

*First a new theory is attacked as absurd; then it is
admitted to be true, but obvious and insignificant;
finally it is seen to be so important that its adversaries
claim they themselves discovered it.*
William James, *Pragmatism*, 1907

Contrary to the common mantra of many authors, oxygen free radicals perform many crucial beneficial roles in sexual function and reproduction. Also contrary to popular claims, antioxidants are not the cure-all for sexual and reproductive problems.

Before becoming a victim of antioxidant propaganda, consider the following facts I have uncovered during my decades of research:

EMODs 42 crucial roles: EMODs (electronically modified oxygen derivatives, formerly called reactive oxygen species, ROS)

EMODs

- modulate vital pathways
- control energy metabolism,
- central component of neutrophil function
- bolster survival/stress responses,
- induce apoptosis,

- manifest inflammatory response,
- regulate oxygen sensing,
- maintain redox homeostasis,
- support fertilization,
- survival kinase activation,
- ion channel regulation,
- apoptosis signaling,
- preconditioning,
- induce necrosis,
- regulate proinflammation,
- modulate the response to growth factor stimulation,
- regulation of metabolism and cytokines
- regulate vascular tone,
- induce the activity of HIF (hypoxia inducible factor)
- signal autophagy,
- generate defense against infectious agents,
- maintain vascular tone,
- control of ventilation,
- regulate erythropoietin production,
- signal transduction from membrane receptors in various physiological processes,
- act as messengers in the regulation of gene expression in development, growth, and apoptosis,
- secondary messengers in intracellular signaling cascades, which can induce the oncogenic phenotype of cancer cells, cellular senescence and apoptosis
- induce a mitogenic response,
- induce cellular senescence and apoptosis and can therefore function as anti-tumorigenic species,
- regulate development and redox homeostasis,
- participate in intracellular signaling,
- regulate "peroxide tone"
- regulate hematopoietic cells,
- regulate vascular tone via activation of guanylate cyclase,
- amplify the immune responses and apoptosis via activation of activator protein I (AP-I) and NF-=B transcription factors in human T cells,
- regulate insulin receptor kinase activity via increased activity of protein tyrosine phosphotases,
- increase expression of antioxidant enzymes and/or glutathione in response to MAPK and NF-kB activation in an effort to restore redox balance, a basal

level of mitochondrial EMOD production appears to be essential for the attainment of a normal length lifespan,

- the level of H_2O_2 affects the expression of at least 80 different genes or proteins, including numerous components of the mitogen-activated protein kinase and nuclear factor kB signaling pathways,

- serve as metabolic intermediates in many biochemical processes including the metabolism of prostanoids, in the regulation of vasotonus, in gene regulation, e.g. activation of nuclear transcription factor kappa B (NF-kB), in the regulation of cellular growth, apoptosis and in the function of intra-as well as inter-cellular signaling and other types of signal transduction,

- modulators in most forms of cell suicide or apoptosis, the signaling cascade utilizes reactive oxygen species (EMODs) as essential intermediate messenger molecules,

- detoxifies pollutants, toxins and xenobiotics,

Here are 42 significant items involving EMODs, which demonstrate their crucial role in homeostasis and disease protection.

– Other than that……

Oxidation reactions are crucial for all plant and animal life, and are a naturally occurring process within the cells. Such systems involve energy production, immunity, detoxification, wound healing, cellular signaling and protection against pathogens and cancer.

Allegedly, EMODs (electronically modified oxygen derivatives, formerly known as ROS, reactive oxidative species) and subsequent oxidative stress have been hypothesized to cause the following damage, relative to sex and reproduction:

- damage of the sperm plasma membrane
- cause a loss of DNA integrity
- lead to a failure of conception
- cause miscarriages
- cause spontaneous abortions
- cause idiopathic recurrent pregnancy loss
- cause hydatidiform mole
- cause defective embryogenesis
- cause drug-induced teratogenicity
- cause oxidant-induced endothelial damage, impaired placental vascularization and immune malfunction

- cause multifactorial and polygenic etiologies of abortion, recurrent pregnancy loss and defective embryogenesis
- cause intrauterine growth restriction and fetal dysmorphogenesis
- oxidant stress has been linked to the formation of antiphospholipid antibodies in the antiphospholipid syndrome
- may even cause childhood cancer
- cause male infertility
- cause sperm dysfunction
- reduce male reproductive potential
- cause endometriosis, ovarian cancer, and polycystic ovary disease via proinflammatory cytokines
- cause male and female infertility, including fetal dysmorphogenesis, abortions, and intrauterine growth restriction
- damage spermatogenesis and Leydig cell steroidogenesis
- cause erectile dysfunction (ED)
- and finally, (and allegedly), peroxidative damage is currently regarded as the single most important cause of impaired testicular function underpinning the pathological consequences of a wide range of conditions from testicular torsion to diabetes and xenobiotic exposure.

One must use extreme care when altering antioxidant defenses. The redox balance is a critical aspect of all aerobic life. EMODs are signaling mechanisms for a vast range of vital metabolic pathways and networks, including those involved in sexual performance. Penile erection is dependent upon vascular smooth muscle relaxation in erectile tissue and penile arteries, the principal mediator of relaxation being the radical, nitric oxide (NO). RMH Note: This free radical response to nitric oxide (NO) can be theoretically blocked by excessive antioxidants.

This book will clarify these assumptions and highlight the role of EMODs in sexuality.

Now, let's have some fun!

Sexual customs in ancient cultures

The sexual revolution of the twentieth century was a substantial change in sexual morality and sexual behavior throughout the West in the late 1960s and early 1970s. One factor in the change of values pertaining to sexual activities was the improvement of the technologies used for the control of fertility. Prime among them, at that time, was the birth control pill.

Rome and Greece

Examination of the structure of social mores of a different time and culture can be fun and enlightening. Today, we likely suffer from post-Victorian values. Today, women do not wear phallic symbols around their neck as a luck charm in the honor of the god of marital fertility nor do we have temples with giant penis statues crowned with flowers.

The Arash's World blog site states, "When in Rome do as the Romans do." This is one of the famous sayings concerning Rome that evolved from a comment made by St. Ambrose to St. Augustine regarding differences in church practices.

Depictions of frank sexuality are abundant in Roman literature and art. The fascinum, a phallic charm, was a ubiquitous decoration. Sexual positions and scenarios are depicted in great variety among the wall paintings preserved at Pomaeii and Herculaneum.

Although the Romans borrowed from Greek culture, literature and religion, even using the Greek language in their aristocratic elite circles, they shunned some of the sexual beliefs that came with them. The idea that the most revered form of love ought to be between two males, mostly an older man with a youth, was not the general consensus among the Romans. This view has persisted throughout time.

It does not mean that homosexuality was not accepted or frowned upon; quite to the contrary, male prostitution was very common and a major source of tax revenue for the Roman treasury. Many of the emperors could not resist these temptations. To the Romans, masculinity was a highly sought-after virtue, and as long as the male was on the giving, and not the receiving end, his masculinity was salvaged.

Promiscuous lovers, like Don Juan or Casanova were the emblem of masculine behavior, but Romans considered it a flaw because it showed a certain lack of restraint. If a Roman male had trouble controlling himself and his urgent needs, he lacked discipline.

In Roman times sex was not given as much importance as has been the case in our post-Victorian sex-obsessed society. Sex was regarded as an every-day necessity, such as food and drink. Therefore, in many cases, sexual acts were committed in plain daylight or within the view of servants. It was much later that St. Augustine had a major say in such matters and sex was seen as something dirty, shameful and sinful.

Marriages were undertaken between families to increase or improve wealth or status and had the purpose of procreation. The "disadvantage" or "inconvenience" of love, especially for the Roman male, was that it might negatively affect a clear head or interfere with rational decision-making.

A curious fact about adultery was that there were cases where it was permitted by Roman society. Slaves were seen as possessions and property, and having sex with a slave was not equated with adultery. Sex with anyone from a lower status was not considered adultery, which conveniently included sex with prostitutes.

Sex was merely an animal instinct, something that emanated from natural bodily functions, and hence, to the Romans, it did not create any kind of obligation or bond between two people.

Valentine's Day was started as rituals involving sacrifices to one of the gods of fertility, Lupercus. In February, which was the month of purification for the Romans, young boys would randomly pick a girl's name from a jar of ballots. Whoever was chosen would become his lover for a year. These traditions were popular with the common people, and it was an early version of matchmaking for lonely singles.

During the same festivities, a goat would be sacrificed, and the hinds were converted into whips with which the priests, and perhaps other males, would randomly inflict lashes on the willing women. That practice, painful as it may seem, was quite welcomed by the female populace, as it was considered to enhance their fertility.

When the emperor Claudius decided to outlaw marriages of soldiers, which he believed demoralized them and interfered with the efficacy of their military services, a priest by the name of Valentine decided to defy the decree and continued to secretly marry the young lovers. When this came to light, Valentine was sentenced to death.

During his prison time he met a jailer's blind daughter and fell in love with her. As legend would have it, on the evening of his death sentence, he passed a note to his beloved which stated, "from your Valentine" and the rest is history. This note-writing practice gained notoriety among the Romans, especially on February 14, so much so that it had to be incorporated and later *Christianized* by the Church.

In ancient Greece, the phallus, often in the form of a herma, was an object of worship as a symbol of fertility. This finds expression in Greek sculpture and other artworks.

Ancient Greek men believed that refined prostitution was necessary for pleasure and different classes of prostitutes were available. Hetaera, educated and intelligent companions, were for intellectual as well as physical pleasure, Peripatetic prostitutes solicited business on the streets, whereas temple or consecrated prostitutes charged a higher price. In Corinth, a port city, on the Aegean Sea, the temple held a thousand consecrated prostitutes.

Rape - usually in the context of warfare - was common and was seen by men as a "right of domination". Rape in the sense of "abduction" followed by consensual lovemaking was represented even in religion: Zeus was said to have ravished many women: Leda in the form of a swan, Danae disguised as a golden rain, Alkmene disguised as her own husband. Zeus also ravished a boy, Ganymede, a myth that paralleled Cretan custom.

India

The oldest evidence of attitudes towards sex comes from the ancient texts of Hinduism, Buddhism and Jainism, the first of which are perhaps the oldest surviving literature in the world. These most ancient texts, the Vedas, reveal moral perspectives on sexuality, marriage and fertility prayers.

Sex magic featured in a number of Vedic rituals, most significantly in the Asvamedha Yajna, where the ritual culminated with the chief queen lying with the dead horse in a simulated sexual act; clearly, a fertility rite intended to safeguard and increase the kingdom's productivity and martial prowess. The epics of ancient India, the Ramayana and Mahabharata, which may have been first composed as early as 1400 BCE, had a huge effect on the culture of Asia, influencing later Chinese, Japanese, Tibetan and South East Asian culture.

These texts supported the view that in ancient India, sex was considered a mutual duty between a married couple, where husband and wife pleasured each other equally, but where sex was considered a private affair, at least by followers of the aforementioned Indian religions. It seems that polygamy was allowed during ancient times. Many cultures practiced polygamy as a way of preserving dynastic succession within powerful ruling families.

The most publicly known sexual literature of India are the texts of the Kama Sutra, which is now perhaps the most prolific secular text in the world. Within certain schools of Indian philosophy, such as Tantra, the emphasis in sex as a sacred duty, or even a path to spiritual enlightenment or yogic balance is greatly emphasized.

China

In the *Book of Changes (I Ching)* a classic text dealing with divination, sexual intercourse is one of two fundamental models used to explain the world. With neither embarrassment nor circumlocution, Heaven is described as having sexual intercourse with Earth. Similarly, with no sense of prurient interest the male lovers of early Chinese men of great political power are mentioned in one of the earliest great works of philosophy and literature, the Zhuang Zi.

Chinese literature displays a long history of interest in affection, marital bliss, unabashed sexuality, romance, amorous dalliances, homosexual alliances—in short, all of the aspects of behavior that are affiliated with sexuality in the West.

The desire for respectability and the belief that all aspects of human behavior might be brought under government control has mandated official Chinese spokesmen that maintain the fiction of sexual fidelity in marriage, absence of any great frequency of premarital sexual intercourse, and total absence in China of the so-called "decadent capitalist phenomenon" of homosexuality.

Japan

In what is often called the world's first novel, the Genji Monogatan (Tale of Genji), which dates back to around the eighth century AD, eroticism is treated as a central part of the aesthetic life of the nobility. The sexual interactions of Prince Genji are described in great detail, in an objective tone of voice, and in a way that indicates that sexuality was as much a valued component of cultured life as music or any of the arts. While most of his erotic interactions involve women, there is one telling episode in which Genji travels a fairly long distance to visit one of the women with whom he occasionally consorts but finds her away from home. It being late, and intercourse already being on the menu of the day, Genji takes pleasure in the availability of the lady's younger brother who, he reports, is equally satisfactory as an erotic partner.

In modern times homosexuality was driven out of sight until it reemerged in the wake of the sexual revolution with seemingly little, if any, need for a period of acceleration.

A frequent locus of misconceptions in regard to Japanese sexuality is the institution of the geisha. Rather than being a prostitute, a geisha was a woman trained in arts such as music and cultured conversation, and who was available for non-sexual interactions with her male clientele. The geisha fulfilled the non-sexual social roles that ordinary women were prevented from fulfilling, and for this service they were well paid. The geisha were not deprived of opportunities to express themselves sexually and in other erotic ways. A geisha might have a patron with whom she enjoyed sexual intimacy, but this sexual role was not part of her role or responsibility as a geisha.

In traditional Japanese society women were expected to be highly subservient to men and especially to their husbands.

The New Testament

The New Testament is quite clear on principles regarding sexual relations. In one of his letters to the Corinthian church, Paul directly answered some questions they had asked about this.

> 1) Now concerning the matters about which you wrote: 'It is well for a man not to touch a woman.' 2) But because of cases of sexual immorality, each man should have his own wife and each woman her own husband. 3) The husband should give to his wife her conjugal rights, and likewise the wife to her husband. 4) For the wife does not have authority over her own body, but the husband does; likewise the husband does not have authority over his own body, but the wife does. 5) Do not deprive one another except perhaps by agreement for a set time, to devote yourselves to prayer, and then come together again, so that Satan may not tempt you because of your lack of self-control. 6) This I say by way of concession, not of command. 7) I wish that all were as I myself am. But

9

each has a particular gift from God, one having one kind and another a different kind."
(1 Corinthians 7:1-9, NRSV)

Ancient Egyptians' Guide to Sex

Much of Our Sexual Health Medicine is Rooted in Practices That First Took Place Thousands of Years Ago

In February of 2012, Sarah Purlackee published the following article in the British Medical Journal. It is available at the website: http://www.medscape.com/viewarticle/757941?sssdmh=dm1.770016&src=journalnl

Introduction

Although we celebrate the progress of genitourinary medicine, how advanced are we in this specialty, compared with our predecessors? Thousands of years ago, did Cleopatra, before engaging in sex with Mark Antony, consider that she should use contraception? Was Antony concerned that the Queen of Egypt might have a sexually transmitted infection? Surprisingly, for this historical couple, the answer to both these questions could have been "yes."

Suited to a Specialty

The topic of reproductive health is not a new concept; several of the papyruses discovered in the ancient tombs of Egypt, thought to be nearly 4000 years old, relate to the improvement of sexual health, mainly in women. (Nunn, 1996)

A common misconception is that medicine in ancient Egyptian times was practiced without logic or understanding of the physiology of the body, and was based on a superstitious religion. The Egyptians were renowned for their medical skills across the ancient world. (Estes, 1993)

In 440 BC, Herodotus, a prominent ancient Greek historian, remarked on the Egyptians' early development of specialist medicine: "the practise of medicine they split up into separate parts, each doctor being responsible for the treatment of only one disease." (Romm, 1999)

The Egyptians' ability to specialize in medical practice came from their advanced knowledge of anatomy, and a good understanding of how the body functioned. Similar to modern medical education, this information was obtained through human dissection. However, such dissection was conducted during the traditional process of embalming (mummifying) the dead.

Sticking to Contraception

The ancient Egyptians understood the importance of the uterus during pregnancy, and recognized the association between coitus and conception. (Estes, 1993)

Although Egyptian methods for birth control are not recommended for modern day use, the contraceptive techniques were not dissimilar from the methods used today.

Many contraceptive techniques involved the ingestion of plant extracts that inhibited ovulation by altering the hormonal balance in the body, much like the modern contraceptive pill. These properties were discovered by farmers, who observed reduced numbers of offspring in cattle that grazed in certain fields. (Haimov-Kochman et al, 2005)

The ancient Egyptians also used barrier methods: "To allow a woman to cease conceiving for one year . . . acacia, dates; grind with one henu (450 ml) of honey, lint is moistened with it and placed in her flesh." (Nunn, 1996)

The lint acted as a barrier against the passage of sperm into the cervix, and honey was used to maintain the lint's position. **Research on acacia has found the tree sap to have spermicidal properties.** (Pakrashi et al, 1991)

Centuries later, contraceptive techniques are still using a similar yet slightly less sticky method, now known as the occlusive pessary or cervical cap, which uses the same principle—a barrier inserted into the vagina in association with a spermicide.

In another contraceptive method, minerals found in the lakes of Egypt were mixed with sour milk. (Morton, 1995)

Modern research has found that the minerals used in this formulation caused degradation of the acrosomal membrane of spermatozoa, a mechanism similar to the chemical nonoxinol-9 that is used in modern day spermicides. (Harayama et al, 1998)

The addition of sour milk may have increased the acidity of the vagina, accelerating the degradation of sperm. **A more peculiar but highly effective intravaginal ingredient was crocodile dung, which was used to deter sexual partners.** (Reeves, 1992)

Pregnancy and the Onion Test

The cessation of the menstrual cycle is an indicator of pregnancy to modern day women, yet the importance of this symptom was not identified by the ancient Egyptians. Despite their lack of knowledge of hormones or female reproductive physiology, the Egyptians did recognize the value of urine testing in pregnancy. According to an article published in *Egyptian medicine*, they were known to believe the following:

"Barley and emmer [wheat]. The woman must moisten it with urine every day . . . if both grow, she will give birth. If the barley grow, it means it's a male child. If the emmer grows, it means it's a female child. If neither grows, she will not give birth." (Reeves, 1992)

When this technique was replicated in a laboratory, a significant number of pregnant urine samples were found to facilitate growth of the barley and emmer. (Ghalioungui et al, 1963)

The accuracy of the Egyptians' observation is impressive, especially since reliable urine tests for pregnancy were not introduced in modern medicine until AD 1929. (Reeves, 1992)

Despite their lack of understanding of the menstrual cycle, the ancient Egyptians' knowledge of the blood supply to the uterus led to the creation of a second and rather radical pregnancy test, guaranteed to bring tears to the eyes of its user. **This test required the insertion of an onion into the vagina.** Should the woman's breath have the odor of an onion on the following day, then pregnancy had been detected. The Egyptians thought that the onion's sulphuric compounds were absorbed into the engorged submucosal vessels in the uterus, resulting in onion breath. (Alaily, 2000)

Unsurprisingly, this test has not been replicated in recent times, but whether this method was an effective pregnancy test remains unknown. An increase in blood flow to the vaginal mucosa has since been recognized as a sign of pregnancy. In 1886, a French doctor described the bluish discoloration of the vagina and labia during early pregnancy, and attributed it to venous congestion, which is now known as **Chadwick's sign**. (Gleichert et al, 1971)

"Weakness of the Male Member"

Although the ancient Egyptians held women responsible for most problems relating to sexual intercourse, they did recognize impotence as a problem arising from men. Egyptian papyruses show records of a prescription for a condition known as "weakness of the male member," involving the topical application of various plant extracts. This prescription was also accompanied by a "magic" incantation, which was to be chanted upon application of the medicine. (Shokeir, Hussein, 2004)

We cannot know whether these remedies had any beneficial effect, although the Egyptians' profound belief in magic might have had a placebo effect on the psychological component of this psychosexual disorder.

Love Bugs

Various texts by the ancient Egyptians have described symptoms of sexually transmitted infections and lice eggs at the base of pubic hairs on embalmed bodies during autopsy. (Morton, 1995)

Common practice was that both men and women would shave almost all their body hair to prevent infestation. In support of this trend, pelvic adhesions have been found in mummified remains. (Aufderheide, 2003)

Some of these adhesions might have been caused by a complication of the sexually transmitted infection *Chlamydia trachomatis*.

Although sexually transmitted infections are thought to have been present in the ancient Egyptian population, they are thought to have had a low prevalence. One reason for this low prevalence might be the stability of the social structure at the time. Dr Joyce Tyldesley, senior lecturer in Egyptology at the University of Manchester, states: "While there are references to gynecological problems, there is very little at all which could conceivably be identified as an STI [sexually transmitted infection]. Clearly, it was not a major health issue."

Despite little evidence, the ancient Egyptians' control over the spread of sexually transmitted infections can be attributed to their marital customs.

Marriage occurred early in life, usually around age 12-13 years; relationships were monogamous; and adultery was considered immoral. (Morton, 1995)

The avoidance of many sexual partners is a form of primary prevention against sexual infections. However, the Egyptians had little knowledge of bacteria and methods of infectious transmission, so this decision probably was not a conscious one.

A Different Battle

The ancient Egyptian civilization is where we find the roots of reproductive science. Although medical treatment occasionally combined religion and science, the Egyptians conducted genitourinary medicine based on accurate observations. Their practices had a poor evidence base by the standards of modern medicine, although recent research shows a strong rationale for their techniques. Some of their theories were flawed, and at times rather extreme, but the medical practices documented in the ancient Egyptian papyruses undoubtedly helped to improve reproductive health.

Historians have accepted that the Egyptian practice of reproductive medicine was more advanced than that in the Western world during ancient times. With the fall of the Egyptian empire, much of their pioneering knowledge was lost. Although the specialty of genitourinary medicine has come a long way in the past 50 years, we should recognize that these modern advances are not as innovative as we might wish to believe.

Secondary sexual characteristics: the female breast

Female Breasts Are Bigger Than Ever, But Under Threat.

In May of 2012, Florence Williams got right to the bosom of her new book in its first line, reeling off names for the most beloved part of the female anatomy: **"Funbags. Boobsters. Chumawumbas. Dingle bobbers. Dairy pillows. Jellybonkers. Nim nums."**

So began William's humorous, but deadly serious treatise, "Breasts: A Natural and Unnatural History."

"We love breasts, yet we can't quite take them seriously," she writes. "We name them affectionately, but with a hint of insult. Breasts embarrass us. They're unpredictable. They're goofy. They can turn both babies and grown men into lunkheads."

Breasts feed us, nurture us and excite us. But the most versatile organ in the female body can also kill us. They are made up of fat and estrogen receptors — so they "soak up pollution like a pair of soft sponges," she writes.

One in eight women will have breast cancer in her lifetime.

Williams, an award-winning science writer, investigates why breasts are assaulted equally by men and a rising number of chemicals in the environment.

She follows breasts through their natural life cycle from puberty to changes during pregnancy, breastfeeding and menopause. And she wonders about their psycho-sexual meaning, writing, "big breasts get a lot of attention."

Breasts are, indeed, bigger than ever, according to her research. The average-sized breast for an American woman is now a C cup and lingerie stories sell sizes from H to KK.

Or, more precisely, the average breast weighs just over a pound, but can double in pregnancy. **The largest (enhanced) breast in the world is 21 pounds or a 38KKK, the equivalent of 2.6 gallons of liquid.**

Williams, 45, was inspired to write the book when she agreed to participate in a study of her breast milk when she was nursing her daughter. The results were startling — her milk was full of chemicals, from pesticides to flame retardants.

"There were reports about toxic and chemical contaminants showing up in breast milk — it was a great way to tell the story first-person," she told ABCNews.com. "I realized there was so much about breasts people don't know."

Today Williams' daughter is 8, and she worries about research that shows girls are beginning puberty and developing breasts younger, perhaps because of exposure to pollutants.

"There are hundreds of chemicals coursing through our blood," she said.

She also explores evolutionary questions. Why do men like big boobs? They are a "sexual signal" that reveals a young woman is mature enough to reproduce. Breasts tend to droop when women age.

But other researchers suggest that the human breast — large and round with a dangling nipple — is unique in the animal world, perhaps to allow the mother to hold the infant in her arms, nurturing the child longer.

"Natural selection versus sexual selection turns out to be a lot more contentious than I expected," said Williams.

Mother's milk is "always the right temperature; it has the correct balance of lipids, proteins and sugars. It is medicinal, nutritious, and, to a baby, delicious," according to Williams.

Her detailed study includes oddities never considered: **Breast milk contains substances similar to marijuana and is sold on the Internet for 262 times the price of oil**, she wrote.

Another interesting factoid: Hour-glass figure Barbie was created by Ruth Handler, a cancer-survivor responsible for inventing the first breast prosthesis in the 1970s.

Women, too, have been obsessed by breast size.

Before silicone, women stuffed their bras with Kleenex and socks, until the earliest implants were introduced in the early 20th century, including glass balls, ivory, wood chips, peanut oil and ox cartilage. Eventually paraffin was used — until it melted in the sun and created lumps.

On the 15th anniversary of silicone implants, **Williams interviewed Timmie Jean Lindsey, who was the first recipient in 1962.**

Now, at 79, she has health problems, including rheumatoid arthritis, an autoimmune disease.

"She told me she was more or less satisfied with her implants, despite the fact that they turned hard, ruptured and she had shooting pains in her chest," said Williams.

In 1976, the FDA began regulating silicone after reports of infections, gangrene and several deaths.

Breast Implants Are Most Popular Cosmetic Surgery

According to Williams' research, an estimated 289,000 women had enlarged their breasts in 2009, the most popular cosmetic surgery. In all, more than 5 million women in the US have implants.

She describes her visit to see a Texas plastic surgeon who performs 800 enlargements a year. She described the clinic as, "Trump Plazas meets Jiffy Lube."

"The plastic surgery industry is masterful at the hard sell," said Williams. "They have convinced women that it's just a simple cosmetic product, like buying a bottle of moisturizer."

Though tempted to try the implants out, she realized, "a lot of perfectly nice breasts ended up looking like water balloons on a skinny rib cage."

In Western culture, breasts are "sexualized to the point where we are having trouble taking them seriously," she said. "Young girls, rather than being in awe of evolutionary miracles, are ashamed of their breasts because they don't look like pornography."

But her biggest concern is the vulnerability of breasts — cancer rates have doubled since the 1940s, according to Williams.

Although Williams can't say with certainty that chemicals in the environment cause breast cancer, she notes that the breast is the one organ in the body that is not fully developed until adulthood — and even the last trimester of pregnancy.

"For many years, the breast cells are undifferentiated and more vulnerable and so are susceptible," she said.

Girls who go through puberty earlier are also at greater risk for breast cancer as adults. "We don't know why," she said.

She notes that in Europe chemicals must be proved safe before entering the marketplace. "We have the opposite and don't take them off the market until they are proven harmful," she said.

Advances in science give reason for optimism, according to Williams. But "government regulatory agencies and the public in general are generally blind to where science is."

"Our bodies are intimately connected to the world around us," said Williams. "If we live in an environment filled with pollution, these things will and do affect our health."

CHAPTER TWO

Begin at the beginning, at the élan vital

The very spark of life is fed by oxygen!

If you put out your free radical, oxidative fire, you extinguish your life!!!

If you douse your inner life-force spark, you smother your élan vital (life force). You can not live without your inner oxidative flame. Antioxidants pose a threat to the oxidative fire within.

Oxygen and its electronically modified oxygen derivative (EMOD) progeny are the *sine qua non* (the essential condition) of man's very existence. **This is an inarguable fact.** Any doubters can prove it to themselves by conducting my "pinch the nose" test. And, it only takes a few short minutes to conduct this revealing test, even in the privacy of your home or office.

Americans are obsessed with medical and health articles, thus making it the third most popular search item on the internet. In fact, the term, "cyberchondriacs" is being used to describe the medically curious. Also, it is well known that we Americans are the biggest "pill-poppers" on the planet.

Even more so, people across the planet are obsessed with sex. Sex even surpasses football as an American obsession.

I have often said, **"Man is the craziest critter on the planet."** To back this up, I had suggested that all one had to do was to turn on the evening news or grab a newspaper. However, if you really want to see how crazy man is, just come with me through the history of aphrodisiacs and sexual prowess.

Without a doubt, a true aphrodisiac would become the hottest drug on the planet, even if it carried a significant down side. But, let's undergo a reality check and scope out the history of these agents that claim to put more "zang in your wang", "zing in your thing" or greater "zippedy in your doo-da!"

The history of medicine is rife with incredulous tales of attempts to cure all forms of ills. Yet, even today, some of these wild approaches still exist as can be gleaned from the following news report of 7-13-2011:

"Ignoring the red-and-white danger sign, Sri Mulyati walks slowly to the train tracks outside Indonesia's bustling capital, lies down and stretches her body across the rails.

Like the nearly dozen others lined up along the track, the 50-year-old diabetes patient has all but given up on doctors and can't afford the expensive medicines they prescribe.

In her mind, she has only one option left: electric therapy.

"I'll keep doing this until I'm completely cured," said Mulyati, twitching visibly as an oncoming passenger train sends an extra rush of current racing through her body.

She leaps from tracks as it approaches and then, after the last carriage rattles slowly by, climbs back into position.

Pseudo-medical treatments are wildly popular in many parts of Asia — where rumors about those miraculously cured after touching a magic stone or eating dung from sacred cows can attract hundreds, sometimes thousands."

Now, let's look at the history of aphrodisiacs.

Let's get current

A Jan 25, 2011 article in Newsweek magazine by Sharon Begley, entitled, "Antioxidants Fall From Grace," cited the following:

A paper to appear in an upcoming issue of the *Proceedings of the National Academy of Sciences* finds that antioxidants might impair fertility. When scientists led by developmental biologist Nava Dekel of Israel's Weizmann Institute of Science applied antioxidants to the ovaries of female mice, ovulation levels plummeted:

follicles released very few eggs. That suggested that ovulation might require the free radicals that antioxidants neutralize. **Further experiments confirmed it:** a type of free radical called reactive oxygen species is produced in response to luteinizing hormone, the physiological trigger for ovulation. That suggests that luteinizing hormone triggers ovulation through an intermediary—namely, reactive oxygen species. **If reactive oxygen species are being mopped up by antioxidants, there's no ovulation.**

Further, Begley (science columnist and science editor for Newsweek) stated, "In 2009, 108 new food products with antioxidants touted on the label reached store shelves in the United States, according to the market-research firm Mintel. That compares with 16 in 2005 and 82 in 2007. "Buyer beware" doesn't begin to cover it."

It is said that slow selling items are flying off of the shelves if the manufacturers stamp the word "antioxidant" on the product.

Here is the party line: Common antioxidants include vitamins C and E. These work by "eliminating" (this is technically incorrect) molecules called reactive oxygen species that are produced naturally in the body. Stress can cause these chemically active molecules to be overproduced and in large amounts they allegedly damage cells indiscriminately. By "neutralizing" (this is also technically incorrect) these potentially harmful substances, antioxidants may, allegedly improve health and slow down the aging process.

None of this has stood up to rigorous scientific scrutiny.

But when Dekel and her research team including her former and present Ph.D. students Dr. Ketty Shkolnik and Ari Tadmor applied antioxidants to the ovaries of female mice, the results were surprising: ovulation levels dropped precipitously. That is, very few eggs were released from the ovarian follicles to reach the site of fertilization, compared to those in untreated ovaries.

To understand what lies behind these initial findings, the team asked whether it is possible that the process of ovulation might rely on the very 'harmful' substances destroyed by antioxidants – reactive oxygen species (EMODs).

Further testing in mice showed that this is, indeed, the case. In one experiment, for instance, Dekel and her team treated some ovarian follicles with luteinizing hormone, the physiological trigger for ovulation, and others with hydrogen peroxide, a reactive oxygen species, EMOD. The results showed hydrogen peroxide fully mimicked the effect of the ovulation-inducing hormone. This implies that reactive oxygen species (EMODs) that are produced in response to luteinizing hormone serve, in turn, as mediators for this physiological stimulus leading to ovulation.

Among other things, these results help fill in a picture that has begun to emerge in recent years of fertility and conception, in which it appears that these processes share a number of common mechanisms with inflammation. It makes sense, says Dekel, that substances which prevent inflammation in other parts of the body might also get in the way of normal ovulation, and so **more caution should be taken when administering such substances.**

Much of Dekel's research has focused on fertility – her previous results are already helping some women become pregnant. Ironically, the new study has implications for those seeking the opposite effect. Dekel: 'On the one hand, these findings could prove useful to women who are having trouble getting pregnant. On the other, further studies might show that certain antioxidants might be effective means of birth control that could be safer than today's hormone-based prevention.'

Dekel and her team are now planning further studies to investigate the exact mechanics of this step in ovulation and to examine its effect on mice when administered in either food or drink. In addition, they plan to collect data on the possible link between females being administered antioxidant supplements and the difficulty to conceive. (Provided by Weizmann Institute of Science)

Aphrodisiac history

Today, all man needs to do is pop down a little blue pill, wait a few minutes and he is ready for sexual action (along with a flushed face, a chance of going blind or having a heart attack). The nuns had always warned the school boys about the direct link between masturbation and blindness. Could they have been right all along?

Aphrodisiacs can include food, herbs, aromas and oils, but they often came from mythic notions rather than practical knowledge. Today, we understand a lot more about the biochemical mechanisms of aphrodisiacs and can thus provide more reliable love remedies.

Darned near anything can theoretically be an aphrodisiac, provided the local culture and mores proclaim it so. More specifically, aphrodisiacs should excite the senses, stimulate the libido and increase stamina–highly subjective factors, to say the least. The term itself refers to Aphrodite, the Greek goddess of love, who could allegedly drive people wild with lust if she wished. Her sacred totem was the sparrow, a bird considered quite randy by the ancient Greeks (the way we consider rabbits randy today). Her followers often consumed the heart, brains or other parts of the sparrow as aphrodisiacs.

But, the fact is that men no longer have to go suck out a sparrow's brain or rip off a rhino's horn or cut off a tiger's penis in order to restore their lost sexual prowess. The fact that rhinos have become an endangered species and are protected from poachers, illustrates the lengths to which man will go, in order to reinvigorate his sexual daring.

Actually, the sex drive is so powerful that it can drive men and women to risk the loss of their families, their livelihood, their wealth, and all of their worldly possessions and prestige, basically everything they have. It happens countless times everyday. Again, just turn on the evening news broadcast.

The overwhelming inner drive creates a nearly uncontrollable desire which must be fulfilled at darned near any cost. It comes down to "screw the sparrow, screw the rhino, screw the tiger, I've got to screw."

Participation in illicit sexual acts has led and continues to lead to broken families and senseless murders.

What biochemical force drives the sex drive? How is oxygen and its radicals involved? Is there any legitimate role for antioxidants in this whole scheme or is this just a "profit thing."

These are some of the questions I will answer in this book. So, let's get on with the history of aphrodisiacs.

An **aphrodisiac** is a substance that increases sexual desire. The name comes from Aphrodite, theGreek goddess of sexuality and love. Throughout history, many foods, drinks, and behaviors have had a reputation for making sex more attainable and/or pleasurable.

However, from a historical and scientific standpoint, the alleged results may have been mainly due to mere belief by their users that they would be effective (i.e., the placebo effect). According to the U.S. Food and Drugs Administration's website, Western medical science has no substantiated claims that any particular food increases sexual desire or performance.

Some purported aphrodisiacs gain their reputation from the principles of a sympathetic magic, for example oysters, due to their shape. But, I am not sure if they are saying it looks like a testicle or if it has tiny labia.

The same factor explains the trade in the phallic-looking horn of the rhinoceros. Other animal-based aphrodisiacs gain their reputation from the apparent virility or aggressiveness of the animal source, such as tiger penis or testicles.

In 7 BC, emperor Cheng died suddenly. It was rumored that he had concubines, who bore him sons, but those sons and their mothers were murdered by the jealousy-driven Consort Zhao Hede; whereas others said he died of a stroke from an overdose of aphrodisiacs, perhaps given to him by Consort Zhao Hede.

The Byzantines made a cake with donkey milk and honey and even Hippocrates, the father of medicine, advocated this fine potion delicacy to liven up one's sexual appetite. The myth of the sexual powers of honey have persisted throughout history, although some consider the whole idea as being debunked long ago.

The Romans and Galen

Aphrodisiac concoctions have been "cooked up" worldwide for millennia. The Roman physician and surgeon to the gladiators, Galen, wrote that foods worked as aphrodisiacs if they were "warm and moist" and also "windy (flatulent)." Examples of such foods were asparagus, mustard and peas. Galen's influence in Europe lasted up until the 18th century.

Spices, mainly pepper, were important in aphrodisiac recipes. And because they were reckoned to have aphrodisiac qualities, carrots, asparagus, anise, mustard, nettles, and sweet peas were commonly considered aphrodisiacs at some point in history.

Today, an aphrodisiac is something that inspires lust. It usually isn't meant to cure impotence or infertility, which are problems that are now handled by separate fields of medicine. But until recently there was little distinction between sexual desire and function.

Any lack of lust, potency, or fertility would have a common cure in an aphrodisiac. Galen thought that a "wind" – or as one 16th-century writer put it, an "insensible pollution" – inflated the penis to cause an erection, so anything that made you gassy would also make your penis erect.

Galen's theories were not the only basis for concocting aphrodisiacs. Mandrake root was eaten as an aphrodisiac and as a cure for female infertility because "the forked root was supposed to resemble a woman's thighs." This was based on an arcane philosophy called the "doctrine of signatures."

Mandrake is a favorite herb that conjures up many superstitious and mythical beliefs, an aphrodisiac among them. You can even find a reference to mandrake as an effective fertility herb in the Biblical story of Rachel and Leah. Marigolds, too, have been looked upon as love potion ingredients.

In fact, marigolds even have a nickname in honor of their sexual properties: "summer brides." Not that marigolds don't have their dark side. In the Dark Ages, women who suspected that they were indeed just "summer brides" and that, come fall, their man would be searching elsewhere, would take marigold seeds and place them into the dirt into which their husband's footprint could be found. It was believed that this practice and only this practice could blind a man's eye for other women.

Cleopatra

Cleopatra was a well known user of aphrodisiacs and she had a legendary sexual appetite that brought empires to the brink of destruction. She supposedly specialized in scents and perfumes, as well as opiates to drug her lovers. Such potions likely contained bear grease, an Egyptian aphrodisiac that has little medicinal value today.

The ancient Romans used many aphrodisiacs, from oysters to frankincense to menstrual blood to the infamous Spanish fly. Some of them had a basis in fact (oysters, for instance, contain lots of zinc, which facilitates male libido), but not all.

A virility-seeking Babylonian in 800 BC, for instance, would cut the head off a partridge, eat its heart and drink its blood.

Oysters may have come to be known as an aphrodisiac because some thought they has a resemblance to female genitals. Few old medical texts listed oysters as an aphrodisiac, although literary allusions to that use are plentiful. This notion is still quite popular in Louisiana.

And, yes, I tried it and it worked for me.

I will discuss oysters subsequently.

We have all heard that oysters are an aphrodisiac, but what about potatoes, skink flesh, and sparrow brains? At one time or another, these things were once considered aphrodisiacs, as was almost everything else that was edible.

Parts of the skink, a kind of lizard, were thought to be an aphrodisiac for centuries. It's hard to say exactly why, but three different ancient authors make the claim. Potatoes, both sweet and white, were once known as an aphrodisiac in Europe, probably because they were a rare delicacy when they were first transplanted from the Americas.

Some aphrodisiacs came out of mythology. Aphrodite, the Greek goddess of love (from whose name, of course, "aphrodisiac" is derived) **was supposed to have held sparrows sacred. We think rabbits are promiscuous animals, hence the *Playboy* bunny and certain lewd sayings** ("screw like a rabbit"), **but the ancient Greeks thought sparrows were especially lustful. Because of the association with Aphrodite, Europeans were inclined to eat sparrows as aphrodisiacs, particularly their brains.**

The Roman poet, Ovid, wrote in *The Art of Love*, after giving a litany of aphrodisiacs, "Prescribe no more my muse, nor medicines give. Beauty and youth need no provocative."

Similarly, some think the only true aphrodisiac is good health achieved by a balanced diet – which isn't all that different from what St. Thomas Aquinas said 800 years ago.

St. Thomas Aquinas, a 13th-century friar, also wrote a bit on aphrodisiacs. Like Galen, he thought aphrodisiac foods had to produce "vital spirit" and provide good nutrition. So meat, considered the heartiest food, was an aphrodisiac; whereas, drinking wine produced the "vital spirit."

Actually, alcohol is one of the few reliable agents known for ages that has any proven effect on sexual desire, even though some claim it reduces actual sexual performance. Its mechanism of action appears to be that it relieves inhibitions and allows for more aggressive sexual advances and contacts.

Therefore, it increases sexual desire by it's psychological effect. In short, for some, it puts them in the mood. However, I believe that the prooxidant properties of alcohol also figure into this situation.

And, yes, I have tried it and it also worked for me.

We do know that overindulgence is said (by modern day psychiatrists) to have the opposite effect on performance, now as in Shakespeare's time. ("It increases the desire but it takes away the performance" comes from *Macbeth*.)

Similarly, coffee is another old contender and it is still sometimes considered an aphrodisiac. Paola Sandroni, MD, a neurologist at the Mayo Clinic, says, "Every time you have an excitation, you have an effect of disinhibition." Also, she reviewed the scientific evidence that exists on many supposed aphrodisiacs, and published her findings in the journal *Clinical Autonomic Research*.

Sandroni believes that calling coffee or anything that contains caffeine an aphrodisiac would be misleading. From my point of view, coffee has to be viewed in light of the fact that it contains both antioxidants and prooxidants, which may cancel out each others effect. Sandroni likens coffee to cocaine and amphetamines because all stimulate the central nervous system (CNS) but have no specific effect on sexual desire.

Sandroni also looked at studies on ambergris, which comes from the guts of whales and is used in perfumes. Some consider the source of ambergris as "whale puke."

Some consider ambergris an aphrodisiac and there is evidence to support this notion. In animal studies, it increased levels of testosterone in the blood, which is essential to the male sex drive, and is thought to play a part in women's libido as well.

Next to oysters (a Louisiana delicacy), the most well known aphrodisiac is the fabled "Spanish fly." It's not just a legend. Such a thing does exist and does have an effect.

Its active ingredient is the chemical cantharidin, which is found in blister beetles. Cantharidin irritates genital membranes, and so it is believed to be arousing because of the urethral irritation.

It's also deadly, causing kidney malfunction or gastrointestinal hemorrhages in people who ingest too much. A quick Internet search is all it takes to find some for sale. Sandroni says she was "horrified" to see how easy it is to buy it.

History teaches us to beware and cautious of aphrodisiacs. Just like commercials for Viagra tell men to beware of any erection lasting longer than four hours, is there any man who actually needs to be told this information?

Older love potions have caused their fair share of pain. **The legend of the famous poet Lucretius has it that his eventual insanity was the direct result of ingesting an aphrodisiac.**

St. Thomas Aquinas

The monk Thomas Aquinas wrote about aphrodisiacs, since issues of the body (and childbearing) were of great importance to the Catholic Church. He applied a more commonsense approach to the topic than Galen, writing about healthy foods which produced "vital spirit."

He also stressed the consumption of red meat and wine, cementing the well-founded reputation of alcohol as a reliable aphrodisiac.

Even the Aztecs and Mayans believed avocados to be *aphrodisiacs* back in *200 BC*. They are rich in the alleged antioxidant phytochemical, glutathione. The California Avocado Commission gathered some psychologists, nutritionists and scientists who found that more than six out of ten study respondents believe eating avocados may encourage feelings of romance.

One might think from the above discussion that combining alcohol and oysters that the effect could be additive. Well, yes, I have tried it also, and it worked for me.

The Puritans

Among the superstars in the world of love potions was the tomato which for centuries was actually known as the "apple of love." Those lusty folks in the south of the European continent were very fond of tomatoes and ate them by the bushel where, in concert with their Catholicism, they produced massive amounts of children; **whereas, the British were so uptight that they discouraged the partaking of apples of love.**

The Puritans latched onto this idea. **The Puritans were so outraged by the alleged sensual properties of the tomato that they conspired to forward the rumor that the vegetable—or is it a fruit—was actually poisonous.** So successful were these founding members of the Religious Right that, like their ancestors today, they were successful in enforcing their morality on the public at large; **tomatoes essentially disappeared from the British diet for a couple of centuries.**

I know of some rural folks who still believe that tomato gravy is a strong aphrodisiac. They say, "It will put some lube in your tube."

Deer antler velvet

Deer Antler Velvet has been prized in Chinese medicine for its use as a sexual stimulant, as well as a tonic. A 2000 year old silk scroll describes the use of deer antler as a remedy for over 50 illnesses. It is considered one of the strongest 'yang', or 'male energy' tonics. Yang energy is an important aspect of sexuality and libido in both men and women, as well as a primary indicator of overall health, strength and vitality. Deer antlers regenerate yearly, and undergo extremely active mitotic growth. One hypothesis of deer antler's sexual enhancing effects, is that these quickly regenerating cells may act in a similar manner to stem cells, and provide 'young and rejuvenating' cellular substance to the body.

Drugs and plants as aphrodisiacs

Certain drugs are considered to be aphrodisiacs. Some of these drugs are Yohimbine, Bremelanotide and a chemical called phenylethylamine or PEA.

Yohimbine

Yohimbine is the main alkaloid of *Yohimbe*. Yohimbe, but not Yohimbine, is often popularly referred to as a "weak monamine oxidase (MAO) inhibitor." Pharmaceutical preparations of yohimbine do not indicate that the drug, which is approved in the US for treatment of impotence (under such brand names as Yocon, Yohimex, Aphrodyne and Viritab), is an MAO inhibitor.

Actually, if MAO inhibition were its only action, I would be against its use because it is recognized as a producer of free radicals (EMODs).

Its main action is as an alpha-adrenergic antagonist, by which yohimbine **may increase genital bloodflow** and both sexual sensitivity and excitation in some people. Preparations of yohimbe bark are available over-the-counter and should be used with caution.

The unrefined yohimbe bark contains several active alkaloids besides yohimbine. Side effects can include rapid pulse, sweating, and anxiety reactions in susceptible people.

Pharmaceutical preparations of yohimbine can also produce these side effects at higher doses, but are available in standardized doses which allow the patient to dose in a controlled fashion. Some patients report a cumulative prosexual effect using the drug over time. It has been around for many years and is frequently advertised in medical journals.

In 2007, investigators studied the effect of yohimbine in the treatment of men with orgasmic dysfunction. They concluded that yohimbine is a useful treatment option in orgasmic dysfunction, (Adeniyi et al, 2007

Yohimbe (Pausinystalia yohimbe)

Yohimbe is derived from bark stripped from a tall evergreen West African tree. Yohimbine, the primary active constituent of yohimbe, is available as a prescription drug, yohimbine hydrochloride, used for erectile dysfunction in men. Yohimbine's mode of action includes blocking alpha-2 adrenergic receptors and increasing dilation of blood vessels. Both of these processes are involved in achieving and maintaining an erection.

The herbal form of yohimbe, has been used traditionally as a sexual stimulant, and has been shown to have similar mechanisms of action as the drug.

Do not use with kidney or liver disease, high blood pressure, or heart arrhythmias. Possible side effects include anxiety, increased blood pressure, and heart palpitations. These side effects are infrequent and reversible.

It is interesting to note that some people who experience adverse effects with the herbal extract have no problem taking the prescription drug.

Other supplements derived from plants that are used as aphrodisiacs, although they have very little or no scientific documentation, include Horny Goat Weed (Epimedium grandiflorum), Muira Puama (Ptychopetalum olacoides), Oats (Avena sativa), Quebracho (Aspidosperma quebracho-blanco), Tribulus (Tribulus terrestes) and Zallouh (Ferulis harmonis). Many of these have been described by Ellen Kamhi PhD, RN.

Bremelanotide

Some compounds that activate the melanocortin receptors, MC3-R and MC-4, are effective aphrodisiacs. One compound from this class, bremelanotide, formerly known as PT-141, is undergoing clinical trials for the treatment of sexual arousal disorder and erectile dysfunction. It is intended for both men and women. **Preliminary results have proven the efficacy of this drug,** however development was briefly suspended due to **a side effect of increased blood pressure** observed in a small number of trial subjects who administered the drug intra-nasally.

On August 12, 2009, Palatin, the company developing the drug, announced positive results (none of the previous heightened blood pressure effects were observed) of a phase I clinical study where trial subjects were instead administered the drug subcutaneously. Palatin is concurrently developing a related compound they call PL-6983.

Bremelanotide is a new drug and so far it appears to be a real aphrodisiac. Bremelanotide increases sexual desire in both men and women.

Melanotan II

Melatonin II, bremelanotide's precursor, has been demonstrated to have aphrodisiac properties. Yet, others claim it has minimal effects.

PEA

PEA, or phenylethylamine, is a chemical present in chocolate. It is the subject of controversy and debate over whether it can be classified as an aphrodisiac.

Chocolate is said to act as a sedative that lowers inhibitions and a stimulant that increases craving for physical contact.

There is some evidence to support the theory that phenethylamine release in the brain may be involved in sexual attraction and arousal, but this compound is quickly degraded by the enzyme MAO and so it is unlikely that any significant concentrations would reach the brain when phenylethylamine is taken orally.

It is also claimed that chocolate contains PEA and is responsible for its aphrodisiac properties.

Fenugreek (Trigonella Foenum-Graceum)

Fenugreek has been recognized as a medicinal plant for centuries. The Egyptians, Greeks and Romans used the aromatic seeds extensively. It was a stable included in the diet of Harem woman to increase the size and roundness of their breasts, and is currently being promoted in several herbal 'bust enhancing' products.

Studies support the practice of modern midwives, as they continue the ancient tradition of recommending fenugreek to improve the milk supply of nursing mothers. Traditional Chinese herbalists used fenugreek for male reproductive issues and kidney problems. It is interesting to note that **in Chinese medicine the kidneys are considered to be the area where sexual energy is stored.**

Although no adverse effects are known, if too much is used during nursing, the urine of mother and child may start to have a maple syrup odor, and could potentially lead to a misdiagnosis of 'maple syrup urine disease.' Fenugreek contains coumarin-like substances, and should be used with caution along with heparin, warfarin and other anti-coagulants. Due to its blood sugar lowering effects, using fenugreek may require a dose adjustment with glipizide and insulin.

(Ho/He) Shou Wu (Polygonum multiflorum)

Ho Shou Wu is usually called Fo-Ti in the US. In China, it is revered for its mysterious properties of rejuvenation and anti-aging, and has been used for over 1000 years as a 'royal tonic' that nourishes the blood, cleanses the liver and kidneys and enhances sexuality and fertility in both women and men. According to legend, it has the unique ability to return grey hair to its natural color. The name He Shou Wu translates to 'Mr. He's Black Hair tonic'.

Polygonum has been shown to improve cognitive function in mice, protect heart tissue from oxidative damage, and has been determined to have surprisingly high estrogen activity, which may account for its reported sexually rejuvenating effects.

Fo ti may have a slight laxative effect, which can be reduced by lowering the dose. One case of possible liver toxicity has been reported.

Arginine

Arginine is an amino acid found in meat, nuts, eggs, coconut milk and cheese. It has many important functions in the body, including the formation of nitric oxide, which increases blood flow to the genitals. Arginine is touted as an 'anti-aging' factor due to its ability to increase strength and lean muscle mass. It is believed to increase sperm motility and male fertility, and may be useful for erectile dysfunction. With higher doses, Arginine is suspected of causing herpes outbreaks in infected individuals.

Lychii Fruit (Lycium barbarum)

Lychii fruit, also called Wolfberry, and Go-Qi-Zi, has traditionally been used in China for thousands of years for its rejuvenating effects on sexuality and fertility. Lychii is a small red berry which is dried and prepared as a tea. Scientific studies have found that polysaccharides found in Lychii fruit allegedly protect both male and female sex organs from free radical damage.

Although adverse reactions are rare, there is one reported case of a possible interaction between warfarin and Lycium barbarum. Lychii should be avoided during pregnancy and nursing, because it contains betaine, which may act as an abortifacient.

Crocin

As per a new study, Crocin has demonstrated the properties of an aphrodisiac in rats. This is supported by pilot tests that demonstrate the efficacy of saffron as an aphrodisiac.

Maca (Lepidium meyenii)

Maca is a cruciferous vegetable like Kale and Broccoli, that grows in the Andes Mountains in Peru. Native people dig up the root-like tuber and brew it into a strong drink. Both men and women partake of this brew shortly before going off in couples for connubial enjoyment. Incan warriors used maca before battle to increase strength and endurance. Laboratory studies have shown a significant increase in sexual function in rodents. There are no reports of adverse effects.

Damiana (Turnera aphrodisiaca)

Damiana has a long history of use as an herbal medicine in Mexico, dating back to the ancient Aztec and Mayan civilizations. Damiana extract contains several chemical constituents, such as flavone glycosides and p-arbutin, as well as the phytosterol, beta-sitosterol. Damiana extract binds to progesterone receptors, which may have some connection to its use as a sexual enhancer.

The species name "aphrodisiaca", refers to the most renown, although not scientifically proven, use of this herb; as a sexual stimulant for both sexes. Damiana was listed in the National Formulary (1888-1947) for menstrual difficulties including headache, acne, insufficient flow, delayed menstruation in adolescent girls, irritability and lack of sexual desire. In Jamaican folk medicine, it is called "Ram Goat Dash Along," because when male goats eat it, their libido appears to increase dramatically!

Ginseng (Panax ginseng)

The name 'ginseng' refers to several plant species. The two most common are Panax Ginseng- called Chinese or Korean Ginseng and Panax quinquefolius- American Ginseng. Chinese and Korean ginseng are actually the same plant species, but differ in the preparation of the root. Korean ginseng is cooked, which turns the root a deep red. It is considered 'hot ginseng' and is the most stimulating form. "Panax" is derived from the Greek word 'panacea' due to the wide range of healing effects attributed to this root. Ginseng confers a youthful vigor to men and women alike. The human-shaped root was called 'man with thighs spread apart' by Native Americans.

The ancient use of ginseng as a sexual stimulant is collaborated by recent studies. The Journal of Urology reported that the "Mean International Index of Erectile Function scores were significantly higher in patients treated with Korean red ginseng than in those who received placebo." While ginseng ingestion appears to have no immediate effect on testosterone levels, other possible mechanisms of action include the pharmacologically active component, ginsenoside-RbI, which increases the secretion of luteinizing hormone(LH) by acting directly on the anterior pituitary gland.

In addition, nitric oxide may be involved in the mechanism of action of ginsenosides on both the central nervous system and gonadal tissues, leading to increased copulatory performance and libido in animal studies. Overall, there is abundant anecdotal and scientific support for the use of ginseng as a sexual enhancer.

Cautions include "Ginseng Over Use Syndrome" which may produce symptoms of insomnia, irritability, anxiety, and heart palpitations. This effect is rare, and most often seen in young men using higher than recommended levels of ginseng. Ginseng use should be monitored by a physician in patients using warfarin, ticlopidine and other blood thinning medications, because it may enhance the blood thinning effects of these medications.

Alkyl nitrites

Alkyl nitrites, (poppers), have a long history of use as a sexual enhancement aid, going back about fifty years. According to the text *"Isobutyl nitrite and Related Compounds"*, many researchers agree that the **alkyl nitrite may be a true aphrodisiac** in the sense of promoting and enhancing sexual response.

The popular recent drugs used to treat erectile dysfunction, Viagra and Levitra, cannot be classified as aphrodisiacs, as they have no effect on mood. They are effective physically but not psychologically.

Perfumes made with natural substances such as almonds and vanilla are said to act as pheromones through the sense of smell, which may add to an aphrodisiac or prosexual effect.

In the United Kingdom, the Intrinsa Testosterone patch has been approved for women with a low libido. Testosterone is recognized as a substance that can boost a women's sexual drive.

Research has shown that women respond with more sexual thoughts and engage in sex more often with the use of Intrinsa. **It is not approved by the FDA in** the U.S. because of increased risk of cancer and uncertainty over long term safety of usage.

Certain rumors and myths abound about particular aphrodisiac combinations and foods. **Mixing Coke and aspirin**, for example, is more likely to cause a stomach ache than anything. Any rumor about it as an aphrodisiac is false.

Foods as diverse as tree bark, shark's fin, hippopotamus snout, chocolate, sea slugs and calf brains have been touted as **aphrodisiacs** throughout **history.**

Another commonly believed aphrodisiac is the consumption of shark fin soup. This food shows no scientific proof for increasing libido. The psychology, or sympathetic magic, behind this practice is that a human is trying to harness the ferocity and strength of the shark. Even today, sharks are being needlessly harvested for their fins.

Few subjects have been so interwoven with folklore and controversy as the effectiveness of aphrodisiacs. The psychosocial complexity of human sexuality, spiritual beliefs and social norms all impact this aspect of human behavior.

The placebo effect may take over when the consumer of certain foods believes they are effective.

In July of 2011, Philippine authorities warned against using geckos to treat AIDS and impotency, saying the folkloric practice in parts of Asia may put patients at risk. Officials have also expressed alarm about the growing trade in the wall-climbing lizards in the Philippines. **An 11-ounce (300-gram) gecko reportedly sells for at least 50,000 pesos ($1,160).**

Geckos are reportedly exported to Malaysia, China and South Korea, where they are used as aphrodisiacs and as traditional medicine for asthma, AIDS, cancer, tuberculosis and impotence.

A health department statement said that the use of geckos as treatments has no scientific basis and could be dangerous because patients might not seek proper treatment for their diseases. "This is likely to aggravate their overall health and put them at greater risk," it added.

CHAPTER THREE

Testosterone

Libido is clearly linked to levels of sex hormones, particularly testosterone. When a reduced sex drive occurs in individuals with relatively low levels of testosterone (e.g., post-menopausal women or men over age 60), testosterone supplements will often increase libido. Approaches using a number of precursors intended to raise testosterone levels have been effective in older males, but have not fared well when tested on other groups.

A French study of DHEA in 280 elderly people, reported in 2000, found **the only benefit was an increase in female libido. A Dutch study found no benefit.**

Testosterone: male hormone, antioxidant facts

Here are a few facts about the **antioxidant "male hormone, testosterone."**

14. It's only known to happen in a petri dish, but Yale researchers showed that **nerve cells exposed to high levels of testosterone were more likely to self-destruct.** The hormone boosted a "cell suicide" mechanism known as apoptosis, which, under normal circumstances, is supposed to help the body wipe out cancerous or otherwise abnormal cells.

And the higher the testosterone level in the dish, the shorter lived the cells were. Exposure to low levels of testosterone, however, had no effect on the cells.

13. *In 2010, researchers halted a study of testosterone therapy in older men because of a higher rate of cardiovascular problems such as heart attack in the group taking testosterone instead of placebo.*

The reason isn't clear, but caution should be used in prescribing testosterone to older men in poor health, Dr. Goodman says. Declining testosterone in men is associated with health problems, but this doesn't mean giving older men testosterone will extend lifespans, he says.

12. Men with sleep apnea are more likely to have low testosterone, and treating sleep apnea can help return it to normal.

But if a man with sleep apnea is diagnosed with low testosterone alone, taking the supplemental hormone can worsen sleep apnea. That's why it's crucial for men with low testosterone to get a thorough workup by an endocrinologist so underlying conditions that can cause low testosterone, such as sleep apnea or pituitary-gland tumors, don't go undiagnosed, Dr. Goodman says.

11. *It has long been thought that taking testosterone increases the risk of prostate cancer. Testosterone treatment can boost levels of prostate-specific antigen, or PSA, a nonspecific marker for prostate cancer, which may lead to more prostate biopsies and more prostate-cancer diagnoses,* Dr. Goodman says.

There are now, however, major questions about whether it's worthwhile to treat—or even diagnose—prostate cancers in older men, given that they're common and often slow-growing.

10. It would be great if an aging man's vigor, muscle power, and sex drive could be restored with testosterone.

But it is not clear whether therapy will do anything for the 75% to 80% of men over 65 who have normal levels of testosterone.

Men with below-normal levels, however, may get a boost in libido, sexual function, and bone mass from supplemental testosterone. And it may help diabetic men with low testosterone build lean muscle mass.

9. Men are often diagnosed with low testosterone after a single test. This is a big problem, says Neil Goodman, MD, an endocrinologist and professor of medicine at the University of Miami School of Medicine.

"If I take blood on a guy and I send it to three labs, I'm going to get three different levels," he said.

Efforts are underway to standardize blood tests. In the meantime, testosterone should be checked more than once, Dr. Goodman says, and done in the morning when testosterone is highest.

8. In men and boys, the right pointer finger is shorter in relation to their right ring finger than it is in girls.

This has even been found in other five-fingered creatures, such as rats. Scientists have found that the difference is a clear marker for fetal exposure to testosterone. **The higher your testosterone level before birth, the lower your pointer-finger-to-ring-finger ratio.**

Men with the lowest ratios made the most money and stayed in business for the longest time, according to the U.K. study of traders and testosterone.

7. **Obese men tend to have lower testosterone than thinner men,** Dr. Dobs says. It's not clear why, she adds, although one possible reason is that obesity promotes a state of widespread inflammation in the body.

"When there's fat cells, there's a lot of inflammatory factors," she says. "**These inflammatory factors have been associated with suppression of testosterone synthesis.**"

6. **In the run-up to a competition, whether it's wrestling or chess, a man's testosterone levels rise,** studies have shown.

After the game, the winner's testosterone will increase even more. **And fans' hormone levels seem to mirror those of their athletic idols.** In a group of 21 men watching a Brazil vs. Italy World Cup match, the Brazil fans' testosterone levels increased after their team won, but the Italy fans' testosterone fell.

5. **In men, taking steroid hormones (antioxidants) such as testosterone as performance boosters can cause testicles to shrink and breasts to grow. For women, it can cause a deeper voice, an enlarged clitoris, hair loss from the head, and hair growth on the body and face.**

In both genders, steroid abuse can cause acne, mood swings, aggression, and other problems.

Men working with an experienced doctor to treat low testosterone or women taking small amounts of testosterone under medical supervision are unlikely to have testosterone-overdose symptoms.

4. Young men who are futures traders get a testosterone spike on days when they make an above-average profit, British researchers found.

And on the mornings when men's testosterone levels were higher than average, their average afternoon profits were higher than on their low-testosterone days, suggesting a possible cause-and-effect relationship.

More experienced traders showed an even stronger tie between testosterone and profits.

3. Men whose levels of testosterone are below normal may lose their spare tire when treated with testosterone.

"Most of the studies show there's a reduction of abdominal obesity in men who are given testosterone," says Adrian Dobs, MD, a professor of medicine and oncology at Johns Hopkins University School of Medicine, in Baltimore.

Because the long-term effects of testosterone therapy have not been well studied, however, **it is generally only recommended in men with below-normal testosterone levels and symptoms such as fatigue, muscle or bone-mass loss, or sexual dysfunction.**

2. Women in love have higher testosterone for the few months after a relationship starts than women who are single or in long-term relationships, a small Italian study suggests.

The opposite is true for men; those newly in love have lower testosterone than men flying solo or with a long-term partner.

As with early passion, though, the changes don't last. **When the researchers tested the study participants again one to two years later, the differences had disappeared.**

I. When most people hear the word testosterone, they think of aggressive behavior.

There is a link between the two—at least in competitive situations, such as with a peer or for a sexual partner.

However, there appears to be a subtler interplay between testosterone and behavior in other types of situations—in both men and women.

(http://health.yahoo.net/articles/mens-health/photos/13-surprising-facts-about-testosterone#0)

According to the **Harvard Medical School Family Health Guide**, testosterone is responsible for men's deep voices, increased muscle mass, and strong bones. It also has crucial effects on male behavior, contributing to aggressiveness, and it is essential for the sex drive and normal sexual performance.

Although testosterone acts directly on many tissues, some of its least desirable effects don't occur until it is converted into another male hormone, dihydrotestosterone (DHT). DHT acts on the skin, sometimes producing acne, and putting hair on the chest but often taking it off the scalp. **DHT also stimulates the growth of prostate cells, producing normal growth in adolescence but contributing to benign prostatic hyperplasia (BPH).**

But while testosterone's effects on many organs are well established, research is challenging old assumptions about how the hormone affects a man's heart, circulation, and metabolism.

A direct association between testosterone and heart disease has never been established, but for many years, doctors have suspected that a link exists. The reasoning goes like this: **men have much more testosterone than women, and they develop heart disease about 10 years before their female counterparts.** Like other muscle cells, cardiac muscle cells have receptors that bind male hormones. Animals that are given testosterone develop enlarged hearts.

Athletes who abuse testosterone and other androgenic steroids have a sharply increased risk of high blood pressure, heart attack, and stroke. And in high doses, testosterone can have a negative effect on cardiac risk factors, including HDL ("good") cholesterol levels.

I believe that athletes are an example of antioxidant overkill, even though they have increased EMODs associated with exercise. In other words, they overcome the EMODs with excessive doses of testosterone and steroids (antioxidants).

The fact that large amounts of testosterone harm the heart and metabolism doesn't necessarily mean that physiological amounts are also harmful. In fact, research is challenging these old dogmas.

It's hard for scientists to study possible new risk factors for heart disease. One reason is that there are so many cardiac risk factors, including family history, age, gender, blood pressure, cholesterol, blood sugar, obesity, smoking, exercise, and personality.

It's also hard for scientists to study testosterone. There is an exceptionally wide range of normal values. Healthy men can have testosterone levels between 270 and 1,070 nanograms per deciliter (ng/dL).

Heart disease and testosterone are mighty complex on their own, and studies that evaluate the two together are more complex still. Scientists who undertake these daunting investigations must account for all the things that influence heart disease and all the variables that affect testosterone.

With all these pitfalls, it's not surprising that more research is needed to fill in all the blanks. Still, even if current information can't tell us if testosterone can protect a man's heart, it can dispel fear that physiologic levels of the hormone are toxic. **Excessive levels of any antioxidant is potentially harmful.**

In high doses, androgens tend to raise LDL ("bad") cholesterol levels and lower HDL cholesterol levels. RMH Note: This is another example whereby over loading of an antioxidant, androgen, is harmful. That's one of the things that gave testosterone its bad reputation. But in other circumstances, the situation is very different.

Men who receive androgen-deprivation therapy for prostate cancer drop their testosterone levels nearly to zero, and when that happens, their cholesterol levels rise. Even within the normal range, men with the lowest testosterone levels tend to have the highest cholesterol levels.

Diabetes is another important cardiac risk factor. **Prostate cancer treatments that lower levels of testosterone produce insulin resistance and increase the risk of diabetes.**

Obesity increases the risk of both diabetes and heart disease. Men with low testosterone have more body fat and more of the abdominal fat that's most harmful than men with higher hormone levels, but since obesity itself reduces testosterone, it's not clear which is the cause and which the effect. **RMH Note: This would tend to argue that obesity is protective against prostate cancer.**

Peripheral artery disease (PAD) is an important form of atherosclerosis in its own right, and it also signals an increased risk for heart disease. **A Swedish study of over 3,000 men with an average age of 75 linked low testosterone levels to an increased risk of PAD.** At present, the hormone does not appear linked to hypertension or inflammatory markers.

As men age, it's not just heart disease they need to worry about. They also begin to lose muscle mass and bone density; red blood cell counts sag; sexual ardor declines; mood, energy, and memory drift down; and body fat increases. In theory, at least, testosterone therapy might blunt or reverse each of these woes. But the theoretical benefits should be balanced against the theoretical risks.

The most serious long-term complications of testosterone therapy include an increased risk of benign prostate disease (BPH). Although some doctors worry that testosterone treatments might increase the risk of prostate cancer, the evidence for this is small. Indeed, **there is evidence that men with low testosterone levels (who therefore might benefit from testosterone treatment) have a higher risk of developing prostate cancer.**

http://www.health.harvard.edu/fhg/updates/testosterone-and-the-heart. shtml. April 2010 update.

Studies in June of 2010 found that **the higher a man's level of natural testosterone, the higher his risk of heart problems,** according to a new study that looked at testosterone and heart disease only in men 65 and older.

"Increasing levels of testosterone were associated with a higher risk of heart disease and death from heart disease," says Kristen T. Sueoka, MD, a resident physician in internal medicine at the University of California San Francisco, who presented the findings at ENDO 2010, the annual meeting of The Endocrine Society, in San Diego.

Dopamine

Illegal stimulants affecting the dopamine system such as cocaine and amphetamines (e.g. methamphetamine, aka crystal meth) are frequently associated with hyperarousal and hypersexuality, though both may impair sexual functioning, particularly with long term use].

Some directly acting dopamine agonists may also cause increased libido, although they can also cause various side effects. **Pramipexole is the only dopamine agonist used in medicine as an aphrodisiac,** and is sometimes prescribed to counteract the decrease in libido associated with SSRI antidepressant drugs. The older dopamine agonist apomorphine has been used for the treatment of erectile dysfunction, but is of poor efficacy and has a tendency to cause nausea.

Other dopamine agonists such as bromocriptine and cabergoline may also be associated with increased libido, as can the dopamine precursor L-dopa, but this is often part of a spectrum of side effects which can include mood swings and problem gambling and so these drugs are not prescribed for this purpose.

The libido-enhancing effects of dopamine agonists prescribed for other purposes has led to the development of a number of more selective compounds such as flibanserin, ABT-670 and PF-219,061, which have been developed specifically for the treatment of sexual dysfunction disorders, although **none of them have yet passed clinical trials.**

Lycium barbarum fruits

Support the folk reputation of L. barbarum fruits as an aphrodisiac and fertility-facilitating agent

Lycium barbarum, a famous Chinese medicinal herb, has a long history of use as a traditional remedy for male infertility. Polysaccharides are the most important functional constituent in L. barbarum fruits. They systematically investigated the effect of L. barbarum polysaccharides (LBP) on rat testis damage induced by a physical factor (43 degrees C heat exposure), on DNA damage of mouse testicular cells induced by a chemical factor ($H2O2$), and on sexual behavior and reproductive function of hemicastrated male rats. The results showed that LBP provided a protective effect against the testicular tissue damage induced by heat exposure. When compared with negative control, a suitable concentration of LBP significantly increased testis and epididymis weights, improved superoxide dismutase (SOD) activity, and raised sexual hormone levels in the damaged rat testes. LBP had a dose-dependent protective effect against DNA oxidative damage of mouse testicular cells induced by H2O2. LBP improved the copulatory performance and reproductive function of hemicastrated male rats, such as shortened penis erection latency and mount latency, regulated secretion of sexual hormones and increased hormone levels, raised accessory sexual organ weights, and improved sperm quantity and quality. **The present findings support the folk reputation of L. barbarum fruits as an aphrodisiac and fertility-facilitating agent, and provide scientific evidence for a basis for the extensive use of L. barbarum fruits as a traditional remedy for male infertility in China.** (Luo et al, 2006)

A wide spectrum

According to Wikipedia, some psychoactive agents such as alcohol, cannabis, methaqualone, GBH and MDMA can increase libido and sexual desire. However, these drugs are not aphrodisiacs in the strict sense of the definition, as they do not consistently produce aphrodisiac effects as their main action. Yet, these drugs are sometimes used to increase sexual pleasure and to reduce sexual inhibition.

Anti-erectile dysfunction drugs, such as Viagra and Levitra, are not considered aphrodisiacs because they do not have any direct effect on the libido, although increased ability to attain and maintain an erection may be interpreted as increased sexual arousal by users of these drugs.

Libido is a function of testosterone and erection is a function of free radicals.

Also, according to Wikipedia, some natural items purported to be aphrodisiacs when ingested or applied to the body are as follows:

- Ambergris

- Arugula (Rocket) (*Eruca sativa*)

- *Atta laevigata*

- Balut (Philippine aphrodisiac)

- Cow cod soup (Jamaican aphrodisiac)

- Borojo (*Borojoa patinoi*)

- Damiana (*Turnera diffusa*)

- Deer penis and antlers (in Taiwan and China)

- Dulce de Leche

- *Epimedium grandiflorum* (Horny Goat Weed)

- *Eurycoma longifolia*

- *Ginko biloba*

- Ginseng

- Kabocha Squash (especially roasted)

- Lettuce, considered an aphrodisiac in Ancient Egypt. Eaten by the sexually potent God of Chaos, Set.

- Maca

- Mannish Water (goat soup, Jamaican Aphrodisiac)

- *Mucuna pruriens*

- Mamajuana Dominican Republic alcoholic sex drink

- Oysters

- Saffron

- *Socratea exorrhiza*

- Spanish fly (catharidin)

- *Tribulus terrestris*

- Yohimbine

Some newly introduced exotic foods often acquire such a reputation, at least until they become more familiar; for example:

- Artichokes

- Bananas. The sap of the red banana is considered an aphrodisiac in Central America

- Mamey sapote (Gabriele et al, 2006). (*Aphrodisiology*: A collection of articles and essays on aphrodisiacs). (*Aphrodisiacs and Anti-aphrodisiacs*: Three essays on the Powers of Reproduction by Johm Davenport).

A 2005 study published in the Guardian UK looked at aphrodisiacs around the world, to see if any actually work. The answer is basically "No."

Although a 2005 study found that amino acids in oysters stimulated the production of sex hormones in rats, there is no evidence that foods like sea cucumber, foie gras or fugu have any affect on levels of lust.

The FDA has stated quite firmly that "sexual enhancement products that claim to work as well as prescription products are likely to expose consumers to unpredictable risks and the potential for injury or even death."

Actually, there are **a few substances that actually work.** The first is Spanish fly, a type of beetle, which when crushed and ingested, irritates the urethra and causes priapism, "a not remotely funny condition in which men sustain an erection for hours." Another is yohimbine, an extract from the bark of a West African tree of the same name. **Unfortunately, its risks are anxiety, seizures and high blood pressure.**

Frog juice (Extracto de Rana)

Frog juice is a beverage revered by some Andean cultures for having the power to cure asthma, bronchitis, anemia, sluggishness and to be a healthy **aphrodisiac** and tonic drink.

The living frogs are killed by banging their heads against tiles. The dead frog is peeled like husked corn.

Frogs are squeezed (in other times and still in rural areas with the hands; otherwise with a household blender) together with white bean broth, honey, raw aloe vera, malt, **maca (an Andean root also believed to boost stamina and sex drive)** and herbs. The resulting frog frappe liquid is a starchy, milkshake-like drink and stings the throat.

Sometimes the frogs are squeezed alive or thrown live into the blender.

The frog drink of the so-called **"Peruvian Viagra"** costs 90 cents. Many Peruvians treat the concoction as their morning and afternoon cup of coffee and the drink is common in Lima.

Female aphrodisiacs

Aphrodisiacs were originally sought as a remedy for various sexual anxieties including fears of inadequate performance as well as a need to increase fertility.

The history relating to the female aphrodisiac goes a long way back to the beginning of mankind. Human body odor is the earliest known aphrodisiac. Scent or the sense of smell is closely related to sexual proclivity as most animal species use scent to determine a female's readiness to mate. Any African animal documentary will attest to this fact.

Pheromones

When a woman feels sexual attraction she may feel a powerful force that draws her to another person. Passionate feelings begin to arise and a longing for this person begins. Human pheromones, natural female aphrodisiacs, are responsible for this incredible attraction. Animals as well as human beings exude a scent that draws others to them. Pheromones have been referred to as "smell prints," that are unique in everyone. Smell is a sense that goes straight to the brain's limbic lobe creating an immediate emotional reaction.

Culinary Uses

Aniseed is a herb that has always been popular for its many culinary uses. It was used as an aphrodisiac by the Greeks and the Romans, who believed it had special sexual powers. It was believed that by sucking on the seeds themselves, men or women could increase their sexual desire. Chocolate and oysters are other examples of some of the many foods in history that have been thought to bring about sexual desire in women.

Chinese herbal medicine has provided us with the most detailed information about aphrodisiacs. However, every culture and society has their own special recipes that are derived from the specific plants and animals that exist in their geographical regions.

Aphrodisiacs come in many forms including animals, plants, herbs, foods, and chemical substances. Ginseng, green oats (avena sativa), mauri, yohimbe, as well as other herbs have demonstrated a strong heightened sexual response in both males and females.

Fantasy

The human brain's ability to fantasize is one of the most powerful natural aphrodisiacs. When a woman fantasizes (about rock stars, football players, fighters, or the guy next door) her brain releases chemicals, electrical responses and glandular substances that act as internal sexual stimulants. A female aphrodisiac can lend a helping hand when the hormone production is low.

Hormone deficiencies

When a woman's body is showing a decline in the output of hormones such as estrogen, progesterone, androgens and testosterone she may notice a difference in her libido. Testosterone (an antioxidant), produced in small amounts by the ovaries, is the hormone that has the biggest affect on the sex drive of both men and women. Hormonal changes can cause a woman's sexual appetite to decrease and result in what may be a devastating blow for those who otherwise had enjoyed a healthy sex life.

Vaginal dryness, painful intercourse and a thinning of the vaginal wall are some of the changes that occur as a result of hormonal deficiencies. Intimacy can become a problem to both the woman and her partner if lack of communication becomes an issue. Her partner may feel responsible for her lack of interest in sex. It is important to discuss the problem and find solutions together.

Sexual empowerment

When it comes to sexual dominance, please remember the old saw, "Women are 100% in charge of sex." So, deal with it guys. You've got to either love it or leave it.

Alprostadil Shows Efficacy in Female Sexual Arousal Disorder

On May 25, 2012, Emma Hitt, PhD published an interesting paper carried on the Medscape website. It was as follows:

A new formulation of alprostadil cream 0.4% (*Femprox*, Apricus Biosciences Inc), administered topically, significantly improved symptoms of female sexual arousal disorder (FSAD) in pre- and postmenopausal women, according to the findings of a randomized, placebo-controlled, phase 3 study.

Irwin Goldstein, MD, director, Sexual Medicine, Alvarado Hospital, San Diego, California, and colleagues presented their findings at a moderated poster session at the American Urological Association (AUA) 2012 Annual Scientific Meeting.

"Female sexual arousal disorder is the second most common sexual health concern, affecting 26% of adult women," Dr. Goldstein told *Medscape Medical News*, "and about 1 in 5 are distressed by the condition, although research in women's sexual health is limited and more is needed."

No product is currently approved to treat FSAD, a persistent or recurring inability to attain or maintain adequate sexual excitement that causes personal distress.

Femprox has been formulated to contain the skin-penetration enhancer dodecyl 2-(N,N-dimethylamino)-propionate, which, according to the researchers, loosens tight junctions of skin cells, thereby enhancing delivery of alprostadil. Alprostadil leads to vasodilation, smooth muscle relaxation, and increased blood flow when applied to female sexual organs.

A total of 387 women were given 10 identical doses of 500 mcg, 700 mcg, or 900 mcg of alprostadil cream or placebo to be used during an 8-week treatment period that was preceded by a 4-week nontreatment baseline period.

Response was measured through the number of satisfactory sexual events (SSEs). Participants were also monitored using the Female Sexual Function Index (FSFI), the Global Assessment Questionnaire (GAQ), and the Female Sexual Distress Scale (FSDS).

SSEs improved with the alprostadil cream at all doses, with a significant improvement ($P = .0002$) observed with the highest (900 mcg) dose (46.3%, 43.5%, and 53.9% for 500 mcg, 700 mcg, and 900 mcg, respectively, compared with 33.1% in the placebo group). The 900-mcg dose also resulted in significant improvements in FSFI, GAQ, and FSDS scores compared with women receiving placebo.

The best efficacy for the cream was observed in patients aged 45 years or younger, Dr. Goldstein and colleagues noted in the poster. In addition, more patients aged 46 years or older reported mild to moderate local adverse events with the 900-mcg dose.

According to Dr. Goldstein, **there are no Food and Drug Administration–approved agents for women with sexual dysfunction**, although several female arousal gels are available over the counter. "The current placebo-controlled trial showed that the active drug versus placebo increased in a safe and effective manner female sexual function using validated measures of female sexual function," he said.

"Women who have female sexual arousal disorder will now have a safe and effective treatment option to improve their sexual function," Dr. Goldstein added. "This medication may benefit a subset of women who are bothered by decreased sexual arousal and whereby enhancing genital arousal will result in improved sexual function."

James A. Simon, MD, a clinical professor at George Washington University in Washington, DC, and president and medical director of James A. Simon, MD, PC, Women's Health & Research Consultants, told *Medscape Medical News* that "whether a woman would be willing to apply the cream to the genital area (clitoris and G-spot) rather than take a pill [off-label: *Viagra, Levitra,* or *Cialis*] remains a significant impediment to use of this preparation."

He added that this study was conducted entirely or primarily in China, and "it is not clear whether women of other cultures (ie, those in North America) would respond similarly or that the interpretation of the rating instruments used (FSFI, GAQ, and FSDS) would be the same."

According to Dr. Simon, FSAD is an important gynecologic problem across the lifespan that increases in older menopausal women. "It may be genital (ie, a vascular condition) or subjective (the sense that there is no arousal even if objectively there is). In the former case, *Femprox* would be an important addition to the available clinical armamentarium."

The study was funded by Apricus. Dr. Simon has disclosed no relevant financial relationships.

American Urological Association (AUA) 2012 Annual Scientific Meeting. Abstract #1498. Presented May 22, 2012.

CHAPTER FOUR

In thinking about increasing oxidative capacity, I tried to think of ways in which we can voluntarily generate EMODs. I came up with the intentional generation of an erection in the male and the erection of the nipples and clitoris in the female.

Thus, is important to discuss erectile dysfunction.

Physiology of erectile dysfunction

http://emedicine.medscape.com/article/1980364-overview

The following was excerpted from an article by Edward David Kim, MD, FACS.

Balance between contraction and relaxation

Andersson summarized some of the information related to the pathways involved in erectile function. (Andersson, 2003)

The degree of contraction of corpus cavernosal smooth muscle determines the functional state of the penis. The balance between contraction and relaxation is controlled by central and peripheral factors that involve many transmitters and transmitter systems.

The nerves and endothelium of sinusoids and vessels in the penis produce and release transmitters and modulators that control the contractile state of corporal smooth muscles. Although the membrane receptors play an important role, downstream signaling pathways are also important. The RhoA–Rho kinase pathway is involved in the regulation of cavernosal smooth muscle contraction. (Chitaley et al, 2001)

Factors that mediate contraction in the penis include noradrenaline, endothelin-I, neuropeptide Y, prostanoids, angiotensin II, and other factors not yet identified. Factors that mediate relaxation include acetylcholine, nitric oxide (NO), vasoactive intestinal polypeptide, pituitary adenylyl cyclase–activating peptide, calcitonin gene–related peptide, adrenomedullin, adenosine triphosphate, and adenosine prostanoids.

Nitric oxide pathway

The nitric oxide (NO) pathway is of critical importance in the physiologic induction of erections. The drugs currently used to treat erectile dysfunction were developed as a result of experimental and clinical work that demonstrated that **NO released from nerve endings relaxes the vascular and corporal smooth muscle cells of the penile arteries and trabeculae, resulting in an erection.**

NO is produced by the enzyme nitric oxide synthase (NOS). (Michel, Feron, 1997)

NOS plays many roles, ranging from homeostasis to immune system regulation. Three subtypes have been identified: nNOS, eNOS, and iNOS, which are produced by the genes *NOS1* (nNOS), *NOS2* (iNOS), and *NOS3* (eNOS). This nomenclature is derived from the sources of the original isolates: neuronal tissue (nNOS), immunoactivated macrophage cell lines (iNOS), and vascular endothelium (eNOS). These subtypes are not, however, limited to the tissues from which they were first isolated.

The subtypes of NOS all produce NO, but various factors trigger and regulate this process. Each NOS subtype may play a different biological role in various tissues.

nNOS and eNOS are considered constitutive forms because they share biochemical features. **They are calcium dependent, they require calmodulin and reduced nicotinamide adenine dinucleotide phosphate for catalytic activity, and they are competitively inhibited by arginine derivatives. nNOS is involved in the regulation of neurotransmission and eNOS is involved in the regulation of blood flow.**

iNOS is considered inducible because it is calcium independent. iNOS is induced by the inflammatory process, in which it is involved in the production of nitrogenous amines. **This subtype has been shown to be involved in the carcinogenic process, leading to transitional cell carcinoma.**

All 3 NOS subtypes produce NO by oxidation of L-arginine, which is one of the basic amino acids. **L-arginine is synthesized from the urea cycle or ingested in food; it circulates in the blood and is found in cells. The concentration of L-arginine within the cell far exceeds that in the circulation. Inside the cell, NOS catalyzes the oxidation of L-arginine to NO and L-citrulline.** Endogenous blockers of this pathway have been identified.

The gaseous NO that is produced acts as a neurotransmitter or paracrine messenger. **Its biologic half-life is only 5 seconds.** NO may act within the cell or diffuse and interact with nearby target cells.

In the corpora cavernosum, NO activates guanylate cyclase, which in turn increases cyclic guanosine monophosphate (cGMP). Relaxation of vascular smooth muscles by cGMP leads to vasodilation and increased blood flow.

Alteration of NO levels is the focus of several approaches to the treatment of erectile dysfunction. Inhibitors of phosphodiesterase, which primarily hydrolyze cGMP type 5, provided the basis for the development of the phosphodiesterase-5 (PDE-5) inhibitors sildenafil, vardenafil, and tadalafil. **Chen et al administered oral L-arginine and reported subjective improvement in 50 men with ED.** (Chen et al, 1999)

These supplements are readily available commercially. **Reported adverse effects include nausea, diarrhea, headache, flushing, numbness, and hypotension.**

Physiology of normal erections

Erections occur in response to tactile, olfactory, and visual stimuli. The ability to achieve and maintain a full erection depends not only on the penile portion of the process but also on the status of the peripheral nerves, the integrity of the vascular supply, and biochemical events within the corpora.

Sexual stimulation causes the release of neurotransmitters from the cavernosal nerve endings and relaxation factors from the endothelial cells that line the sinusoids. **NOS produces NO from L-arginine. This, in turn, produces other muscle-relaxing chemicals such as cGMP and cyclic adenosine monophosphate (cAMP), which work via calcium channel and protein kinase mechanisms.**

This results in the relaxation of smooth muscle in the arteries and arterioles that supply the erectile tissue, producing a dramatic increase in penile blood flow.

Relaxation of the sinusoidal smooth muscle increases its compliance, facilitating rapid filling and expansion (40-52% of the corpora cavernosa tissue is composed of smooth muscle cells). The venules beneath the rigid tunica albuginea are compressed, resulting in near-total occlusion of venous outflow. These events produce an erection with an intracavernosal pressure of 100 mm Hg.

Additional sexual stimulation initiates the bulbocavernous reflex. The ischiocavernous muscles forcefully compress the base of the blood-filled corpora cavernosa, and the penis reaches full erection and hardness when intracavernous pressure reaches 200 mm Hg or more. At this pressure, both the inflow and outflow of blood temporarily cease.

Detumescence results from the cessation of neurotransmitter release, the breakdown of second messengers by PDEs, and sympathetic nerve excitation during ejaculation. Contraction of the trabecular smooth muscle reopens the venous channels, allowing the blood to be expelled, which results in flaccidity.

Pathophysiology

Penile erections involve an integration of complex physiologic processes involving the CNS, peripheral nervous system, and hormonal and vascular systems. Any abnormality involving these systems, whether from medication or disease, has a significant impact on the ability to develop and sustain an erection, ejaculate, and experience orgasm.

ED is often associated with other vascular diseases and conditions such as diabetes, hypertension and coronary artery disease.

Other conditions associated with ED include neurologic disorders, endocrinopathies, benign prostatic hyperplasia, and depression.

Vascular diseases

Vascular diseases account for nearly half of all cases of ED in men older than 50 years. Vascular diseases include atherosclerosis, peripheral vascular disease, myocardial infarction, and arterial hypertension.

Vascular damage may result from **radiation therapy to the pelvis and prostate in the treatment of prostate cancer.** (Valicenti et al, 2002)

Both the blood vessels and the nerves to the penis may be affected. Radiation damage to the crura of the penis, which are quite susceptible to radiation damage, can induce ED. **Data indicate that 50% of men undergoing radiation therapy lose erectile function within 5 years after completing therapy.** Fortunately, some tend to respond to one of the phosphodiesterase-5 (PDE-5) inhibitors.

CHAPTER FIVE

My philosophical approach (Excerpted from my book: *Heart Disease and Antioxidant Failures*)

In many ways, we are creatures modulated by our biochemical instincts and unable to change our physiological destinies. Instincts of individual cells rapidly discuss their collective needs and sort through ingested food stuffs accordingly; normally, assimilating the essentials and discarding the un-needed.

Small dietary changes will make little difference. Please remember that a hungry belly gives a human permission to violate any dietary regimen; in the animal world, it is a license to kill or cannibalize.

Our fatal flaw has been to believe that we can readily and easily change our biochemical signatures, only to be reminded that it is chiseled in cytoplasmic stone. Our attempts to alter our fates have always come back to bite us in our presumptuous posteriors.

Our perceived successes are only temporary illusory mirages, arising from the dying thirst of trying to do better but which nature interprets as trying to interfere.

Instinct, the puppeteer, will ultimately pull most of the strings of life, which have been woven by genetics into the environmental fabric. Compulsive attempts at controlling our destinies are an arduous, dangerous and at times, perhaps a futile evolutionary reflex. Ergo, we see the fanaticism of carbohydrate, fat or protein dieting.

We fantasize of a singular magic pill which is capable of giving us broad disease protection and of correcting wide ranging pathophysiologies. Indeed, this is only a dream world. Today, Pharma's middle name is "harm."

We are a map of intertwined, twisting and writhing biochemical pathways and a cloudy condensate of speeding, blurred subatomic particles. The continent of the body is ruled by the smallest of molecular species, electronically modified oxygen derivatives (EMODs).

EMODs are not biological nomads but are tried and true travelers of the body's cellular, tissue and organ mosaics. As such, the tactician, hydrogen peroxide is allowed to roam the intracellular wilderness and extracellular expanse at will. Singlet oxygen and its brethren serve as sentries and protoplasmic protectors, by affecting neoplastic apoptotic execution and carrying on all important intercellular chatter.

All chemical radicals have two faces, one for giving and one for taking, one for oxidation and one for reduction. The metabolic mirror has the face of the other radical twin peering through from behind it, which conveniently lends itself to alternating oxidative states. Survival is about moral indifference and curing disease is about capitalization on opportunity and intellect utilization.

Today's scientific papers are filled with "fuzzy math and statistical chicanery" in attempts to garner some semblance of insight into the biochemically mysterious cell. At times, it appears that we are willing to accept erroneous theories, if it will allow us to remain affixed to the governmental grant-teat for prolonged feeding.

At other times, we appear to have thought paralysis. However, we must speak and question with impunity and not be afraid to put a suffocating foot onto the neck of another's misguided theory. In a world of 25,000 journals, spewing out over a million papers per year, their collective pseudo-scientific-vomitus rarely passes the smell test of veracity or the common sense test of intellectual clarity.

Investigators fill pages with hyperbolic verbiage and fabricated charts and tables to support their myopic viewpoint, whilst readily ignoring the obvious. Nothing could be more illustrative of this nonsensical situation than the incrimination of oxygen as being a ruthless killer of aerobes and biota. Common sense has been silenced by nonscience/nonsense.

I believe that the free radical theory of oxidative stress and aging has outlived its time of usefulness and now serves only as a decaying red herring to obfuscate scientific truth. This is particularly true in the trumped up case of a cause and effect relationship between lipoprotein-cholesterol oxidation and cardiovascular disease, atherosclerosis and plaque formation. The chemical kings-of-spin have convinced hordes of scientists that oxidative stress is "for real."

Basically, I can sum up the data concerning free radicals and disease causation in the following few words: "The literature is chock-full of conflicting, inconsistent and confusing data, which is frequently presented as absolute truths handed down by the man behind the opaque curtain of scientific confusion."

Researchers frequently lack the ability to see their results clearly and they paint over their studies with a translucent film of cheap mathematical make-up to hide their "investigative imperfections." Yet, they hawk their faux-facts to stir up an internal civil war between the dark force of oxidation and the beneficent battalions of antioxidants. All the while, the so called battle between oxidants and antioxidants is only a war in a calculated world of perception. It is "the war that never was."

There is no classic war game between free radicals and antioxidants.

In fact, oxidants frequently require an antioxidant for the donation of an electron. In other words, you could not form as many EMODs without the electron contributions from antioxidants.

The metabolic and disease predictive power of antioxidant criteria must be validated in clinical trials before it can be accepted. This has not happened. In fact, there is no predictive ability associated with the free radical theory of oxidative stress and aging.

Simply put, the free radial theory has failed to meet the criteria of the scientific method.

Following years of intense investigation of the scientific literature, I now have "greater clarity and reduced uncertainty" about the impact of oxygen free radicals with the living/breathing cell. The risks of unnatural EMOD (electronically modified oxygen derivatives) reduction, with antioxidants (scavengers, traps, quenchers, etc.), may well be greater than previously thought.

I believe that there exists a "tipping point or trigger point" at which especially low EMOD levels (an EMOD insufficiency) allows for uncontrolled cellular proliferation. Data from immunosuppressed patients clearly supports my view.

Thus, there is a need for real concern.

Double blind randomized controlled human studies (RCTs) started to indicate that the potential for antioxidant harm was a slumbering giant. I believe that the **"antioxidant behemoth"** has now been awakened, as indicated by increased risks for cancer, atherosclerosis, strokes and overall mortality, which is currently linked to antioxidants. I feel that we are experiencing an antioxidant overload because of the antioxidant supplements, fortified foods and synthetic antioxidant preservatives in a wide array of foods, which ultimately become strewn throughout the environment and food chain and can be ingested or eaten.

I believe that, in general, we fail to appreciate the fact that we swim beneath and within a sea of di-radical oxygen molecules, which constantly bathes all external and most internal parts of our being. One in every five atmospheric molecules is an oxygen molecule. We are continually immersed in this ocean of di-radical oxygen.

Thus, I do not accept the customary hoopla concerning the killer-toxicity of oxygen radicals.

Additionally, I have written about the occurrence of bacterial vegetations on scarred or artificial heart valves and that I believe that the inability of these prosthetic valves to protect themselves with EMOD generation leads to the appearance of the bacterial growth.

I now further believe that a similar situation is responsible for the commonly recognized situation in which prosthetic materials surgically introduced into the body are a nidus (center or location) for infection. These prosthetic materials have a total lack of or an insufficiency of EMODs, because they can not produce them and consequently, they "allow" the development of bacterial infections and calcium deposition.

The scientific literature is replete with references to oxidation or radicals as being damaging or deleterious. This is the direct effect of the flawed "Free Radi-crap theory" (my sardonic term for the free radical theory) and to its nigh carte blanche acceptance by the medico-scientific community. The biased history of free radicals illustrates this point clearly. (Davies et al, 2005).

Several therapeutic strategies have been recommended to slow the early atherosclerotic process in asymptomatic subjects in order to reduce the risk of cardiovascular events. Additional steps proposed to possibly slow the atherosclerotic process have included interventions to decrease newly emerging coronary risk factors, such as oxidative stress (these have failed thus far) and inflammation (accumulating data is also failing here).

Consuming a diet rich in fruits and vegetables provides antioxidant vitamins, and carotenoids, which were believed to inhibit tissue damage derived from oxidative processes and were believed to slow the progression of early atherosclerosis, modify the increase in carotid intima media thickness and, consequently, reduce cardiovascular events. **Thus far, the supplemental vitamin studies have basically been failures, in that the antioxidants are either frequently ineffective or they cause many adverse effects, including death.**

Even the overly-hyped beneficial contribution of fresh fruits and vegetables is being scientifically questioned.

It is my belief that plaques form at locations of EMOD insufficiencies. I believe that oxidation of microaggregates would allow for their excretion. Thus, heart valves, with high fibrous content and valve prostheses, with no ability to produce EMODs, should be at high risk for infections, calcification or plaque formation (and they are).

The height of "unintended consequences"

My prior studies show that the antioxidant vitamins A, C & E can produce, the height of "unintended consequences."

Some antioxidant harmful conclusions from my book, *"Death In Small Doses?"*:

- Antioxidant vitamins cause harm…widespread harm
- They increase risk of various forms of heart disease, i.e., heart failure, ischemia, non fatal myocardial infarction
- They accelerate atherosclerosis and plaque formation
- They increase the risk of common cancers, such as breast, prostate and lung
- They increase total mortality

- They increase stroke mortality
- They increase risk of bone fractures
- They increase disease risks for smokers, diabetics and those exposed to asbestos
- They increased the risk of falling
- They increased the risk of low-birth-weight babies
- They increased the risk of gestational hypertension
- They damage sperm DNA
- They do not perform as advertised in keeping disease at bay
- They do not prevent aging
- They shorten life span, due to increased mortality and disease incidence
- They are not recommended by the vast majority of major medical and scientific organizations
(Howes, Book I, 2010) (Howes, Book 2, 2010)

My book serves as a cautionary tale about the myths and potential risks related to dietary supplements and makes the point that more is not necessarily better. We know that **vitamin C prevents scurvy, vitamin D prevents rickets, and thiamine will prevent beriberi.**

However, this in no way means that in a well-nourished population, these supplements will prevent the chronic diseases, cardiovascular diseases, cancer, and other chronic diseases of the 20th and 21st centuries, or that more will be better.

Ad libitum use of multivitamins does not reduce all-cause mortality in women; to the contrary, it slightly increases it. In a 2011 by Mursu et al study, the Iowa Women's Health Study, more than 38,000 women who were, on average, age 62, were followed for up to 22 years. **Multivitamins, vitamin B6, folic acid, iron supplements, copper, and zinc were all associated with some increase in mortality risk.** In replication analyses in later follow-up periods, **excess risks continued to be seen with iron supplements.** (Mursu et al, 2011)

The title to this article should have read: **Vitamin Supplements Associated With Increased Risk For Death.**

Mursu et al stated, "Although we cannot rule out benefits of supplements, such as improved quality of life, our study raises a concern regarding their long-term safety."

We know from randomized trials that many of the antioxidant vitamins, in fact, increase risks, especially in well-nourished populations.

The randomized trials of beta-carotene and vitamin E have not shown clear health benefits but instead, studies have shown increased risks, such as increased risk of prostate cancer.

In fact, many say that there is no reason for otherwise healthy men to take vitamin E. (Baker et al, 2011)

Laurence H. Baker, DO, professor of internal medicine and pharmacology at the University of Michigan, Ann Arbor, agrees that his findings were unexpected.

"Vitamin E doesn't prevent prostate cancer; it doesn't prevent any cancer, despite the claims of some, and it doesn't promote cardiovascular health, despite the claims of many." he said in an interview.

"There is no evidence to support any of these claims, yet thousands or even millions of men include vitamin E in their supplementation," Dr. Baker continued. "What this tells us is that even though we assume something to be good, it may not be. In fact, it may be harmful. The assumption is that because vitamin E is an antioxidant, it's good for us. But that isn't the case."

We know that beta-carotene increases lung cancer risk in smokers, and vitamin E was recently linked to an increased risk for prostate cancer in men and was previously linked to an increased risk for hemorrhagic stroke.

Well-nourished populations do not appear to derive any benefits from these supplements.

Also, in some cases, there appears to be a U-shaped curve where risk is increased with low-intake deficiency states as well as with high intake.

Overall, for most vitamins and minerals, a balanced diet will provide adequate intake.

A prudent statement is that, "polynutrient" is far less toxic than polypharmacy.

In addition to the 500+ studies showing the ineffectiveness of antioxidants, there are now over 170 showing their harmful effects. I presented these in my 2012 book entitled, *Antioxidants Linked to Deadly Unintended Consequences*.

In summary, scientific testing of some antioxidant study reports have selectively shown the following:

Antioxidants have increased mortality by as high as 17% and 19%.

Antioxidants have increased lung cancer by 18% and 28%, esophageal cancer deaths by 14% and 22.1%, breast cancer by 19%, hemorrhagic stroke deaths by 50%, ischemic heart disease by 11%, and cardiovascular disease by 18%.

Vitamin E increased risk of prostate cancer by 17%.

Antioxidants have increased prostate cancer deaths, elevated the risk of squamous cell carcinoma, doubled the risk of adenoma recurrence, increased the rate of second primary cancers, and increased recurrence of head and neck tumors.

Antioxidants increased the incidence of melanoma in women by 4 fold. (Hercberg et al, 2007, VITAL)

Patients taking an antioxidant were 1.65 times more likely to suffer a return of their original cancer.

Three major studies were stopped early due to unexpected harmful outcomes and adverse effects for study participants: ATBC, CARET and SELECT. (Heinonen et al, 1994, ATBC) (Omenn et al, 1996, CARET) (Lippman et al, 2009, SELECT) respectively.

Antioxidants have increased ischemic heart disease, deaths from fatal coronary heart disease, increased risk of nonfatal and fatal myocardial infarction, decreased platelet function, increased intima-to-media thickness, negated statin effects, increased risk of hospitalization for heart failure and hypertension, altered liver function tests, increased blood pressure, and increased blood loss after cardiac surgery.

Antioxidants have increased hemorrhagic stroke deaths as much as 22% to 50%, increased risk of subarachnoid hemorrhage 50% and increased risk of intracerebral hemorrhage 62% and increased risk of fatal subarachnoid hemorrhage 181%.

Antioxidants have increased wheezing, productive coughs, and risk of asthma.

In diabetics, antioxidants have increased pre-diabetic changes in glucose metabolism, increased severity of diabetic retinopathy, and increased blood pressure.

Antioxidant have increased preterm deliveries, premature rupture of membranes and low birth weight, increased gestational hypertension, increased risk of hospitalization, altered liver function tests, increased risk for severe preeclampsia, and fetal loss or perinatal death in women at risk for preeclampsia.

Antioxidants have increased risk of tuberculosis by 72% and pneumonia by 14%, indicating an altered immune system.

Antioxidants have adversely affected muscle performance and hampered endurance capacity.

Antioxidants increased risk of cataracts by 38% and by 56% in hormone replacement users, and increased risk of age-related macular degeneration (AMD).

Antioxidants increased the risk of hip fractures, damaged sperm DNA, increased epistaxis (nose bleed) and mother to child transfer of HIV.

Other than that…..

Cancer related harmful effects of antioxidants: (new findings as of 10-29-11)

Antioxidants BHA and BHT increase carcinogenesis in animal studies.

The antioxidant, genistein, can cause chromosomal aberrations and DNA damage, in sperm and lymphocytes.

Genistein (an antioxidant) enhances growth of breast cancer cells in vitro.

Supplementation studies indicate soy may promote breast cancer development.

Combinations of antioxidants C and E may cause sperm damage.

Genistein (an antioxidant) induces DNA breaks in human tumor cell line and induced mitogenesis in mouse tumors.

Lycopene (an antioxidant) facilitated invasion of prostate cancer cells in vitro.

Selenium increased basal cell, squamous cell and total nonmelanoma skin cancer (NPC Trial).

Genistein (an antioxidant) enhanced tumor development of estrogen-dependent cells treated with carcinogens.

Genistein (an antioxidant) blocked the chemotherapy drug, tamoxifen, and attenuates its anti-tumor effect.

Vitamin E caused DNA damage in African-American men.

Excessive multivitamin use increased risk of fatal prostate cancers.

Vitamin E increased risk of oral premalignant lesions.

Genistein (an antioxidant) increased genomic instability of mouse lymphoma cells.

Genistein (an antioxidant) can reverse the cancer-inhibitory effect of anti-tumor agents.

Polymorphisms of the antioxidant enzyme, GPxI, increase risk of cancer.

Selenium (an antioxidant) can enhance mutagenesis and chromosomal abnormalities.

Genistein (an antioxidant) caused teratogenic effects in zebra fish embryos.

Alpha-tocopherol (vit E) increased adenocarcinomas of mammary glands in rats.

Carotenoids (an antioxidant) increased the risk of dying from cancer in women.

Genistein increased aromatase in human adrenocortical cancer in rats.

Neither the American Cancer Society nor the American Institute for Cancer Research recommend any dietary supplement for preventing cancer or cancer recurrence.

Other harmful effects of antioxidants:

Vitamin E and C slowed greyhound dogs.

Vitamin E made respiratory infections more severe.

Glutathione peroxidase (GPxI) interfered with insulin function and caused glucose intolerance.

Genistein produced a wide range of reproductive biological and behavioral defects in rats.

Vitamin C combined with grape seed extract increase systolic BP and diastolic BP.

Alpha-tocopherol caused an unexpected increase in cholesterol levels.

Thirteen percent (13.3%) of supplement users attributed adverse effects to multivitamins/multiminerals.

Alpha-tocopherol (and mixed tocopherols) increased systolic and diastolic BP and pulse pressure and heart rate, esp. in type 2 diabetes patients.

Vitamin A increased mother-to-infant risk of transmission of HIV.

Selenium increased risk of type 2 diabetes.

Post-exercise antioxidants negated good effects on lowering BP and vasodilation.

Antioxidants appear to hinder pos-exercise recovery of muscle damage.

The casual use of vitamins C and E are not recommended for athletes.

Vitamin A increased risk of acute respiratory infection.

Vitamins A and C increase risk of gestational hypertension and low birth weights of neonates (newborns).

Bisphenol A (BPA, an antioxidant) decreased semen quality and increased sperm DNA damage.

Multivitamin/minerals caused third trimester women to experience preterm birth.

Selenium over use causes a wide range of effects, including fatigue and hair loss.

Soy products, isoflavones and genistein has implications for testicular malfunction in neonates.

Fats found in fish oil can block chemotherapy drugs in mice.

Taking supplements increased the risk of dying by 2.4% in women.

Vitamin E and beta-carotene increased risk of age-related macular degeneration.

BPA before birth negatively affected girl's behavior at age 3.

Use of multivitamins, B6, folic acid, magnesium, zinc, iron and copper increased risk of all-cause mortality.

Additionally, over 500 scientific studies have reported on the ineffectiveness of the antioxidants. They also indicate that unless there is a proven deficiency state, these antioxidants are unnecessary and dangerous. Further, the antioxidants in supplements do not work as effectively as those found in fresh fruits and vegetables.

CHAPTER SIX

Organizations not recommending antioxidant vitamins

The following organizations or groups either DO NOT RECOMMEND antioxidant vitamins or have found inconclusive evidence of their benefit:

- The American Heart Association (AHA)
- The American College of Cardiology
- American College of Cardiology Foundation Task Force on Clinical Expert Consensus Documents
- The American College of Cardiology/American Heart Association Task Force on Practice Guidelines
- The AHA Scientific Position of the American Heart Association
- The American Heart Association Atherosclerosis, Hypertension, and Obesity in Youth Committee, Council of Cardiovascular Disease in the Young, With the Council on Cardiovascular Nursing
- Scientific Statement From the American Heart Association and the American Diabetes Association
- National Heart Foundation of Australia's Nutrition and Metabolism Advisory Committee
- The 2006 AHA Diet and Lifestyle Recommendations
- The American Cancer Society
- The American Diabetes Association
- The National Cancer Institute (NCI)
- Institute of Medicine of the National Academies
- National Academy of Sciences
- The American Academy of Family Physicians
- The U.S. Food and Drug Administration (FDA)

- Food and Nutrition Board, Institute of Medicine
- The Food and Nutrition Board of the National Academy of Sciences
- United States Preventive Services Task Force (USPSTF)
- The American College of Chest Physicians (ACCP)
- National Institutes of Health State-of-the-Science Conference
- The American Cancer Society Guidelines on Nutrition and Physical Activity for Cancer Prevention
- The Swedish Council of Technology Assessment
- The Medical Letter
- National Heart Foundation of Australia's Nutrition and Metabolism Advisory Committee
- The Oregon Health and Science University
- The Canadian Task Force on Preventive Health Care (CTFPHC)
- Food Standards Agency/ the British Nutrition Foundation (BNF)
- The Nutrition Committee of the American Heart Association Council on Nutrition, Physical Activity, and Metabolism
- Quackwatch
- The Physicians Health Study
- The 2008 VITAmins and Lifestyle (VITAL) study
- The Physicians' Health Study II Randomized Controlled Trial

(Howes, Am J Cos Surg. 2009) (Howes, Book 1 & 2. 2010).

TEN KEY LIES DOMINATE THE MAINSTREAM MEDIA

Lie #1 - Antioxidant vitamins are completely safe and free from harm

Lie #2 - There have never been any deaths attributable to any of the antioxidant vitamins

Lie #3 - The antioxidant vitamins can cure, reverse or prevent cancer

Lie #4 - The antioxidant vitamins can cure, reverse or prevent heart disease

Lie #5 - The antioxidant vitamins can cure, reverse or prevent strokes

Lie #6 - The antioxidant vitamins will increase your life span and prevent aging

Lie #7 - The antioxidant vitamins can cure, reverse or prevent eye diseases, such as cataract formation or macular degeneration

Lie #8 - Oxygen free radicals are toxic and lethal

Lie #9 - Oxidation is destroying cells by blowing holes in them

Lie #10 - (and THE BIGGEST WHOPPER OF ALL):

Oxygen is killing all of us and will bring death to all humans!

TEN THINGS YOU ARE NOT SUPPOSED TO KNOW ABOUT ANTIOXIDANT VITAMINS

#1 - They are not tested by federal agencies for safety or efficacy

#2 - Hundreds of studies show their ineffectiveness (over 250)

#3 - They can not prevent or cure cancer

#4 - They can not prevent or cure heart disease

#5 - They can not prevent or cure strokes

#6 - They can not prevent or cure eye diseases

#7 - They do not increase the life span or prevent aging and they may increase overall mortality

#8 - Over eighty scientific studies have shown their wide ranging harmful effects

#9 - Oxygen free radicals are of low toxicity and essential for normal metabolism

#10 - Oxygen is our most essential ally in sustaining a healthful condition, in fighting pathogens and in killing cancer cells

Basically, the antioxidant vitamins are today's snake oil. They have unknown benefits with known harmful effects. Patient safety, and not profits, should always be the priority.

MY GRAND OPENING

"It is better to appear stupid than to open your mouth and remove all doubt."
-Mark Twain

But, here goes anyway!

The support of the establishment for antioxidant use is misleading and flawed. The scientific evidence leaves one with disdain and contempt against powerful advertising forces.

When the drug companies come out and admit to "some bad risk" from deadly drugs or supplements, you know that "the whole truth" is actually much worse.

At first sight, the magnificent claims by antioxidant proponent suppliers in heart disease, infection and cancer appear astonishing. However, their aloofness is quickly abolished by the reality of the data itself.

When science confirms just one of my ideas, people will understand why I was prepared to stake my scientific reputation on the medical significance of oxygen and its electronically modified derivatives (EMODs).

If my book doesn't shock you, either you haven't understood it or *you have not been paying attention.* Please focus.

My book will educate you on all you need to know about redox (reduction/oxidation) chemistry and all your doctor needs to know….**but probably doesn't.**

I discuss forthrightly controversies that organized medical science would prefer to ignore. They prefer to accept the flawed free radical theory, ignore the data and simply move on.

The scientific understanding of radicals has not yet led to any therapeutic application. (Wingler, Schmidt, 2009).

That needs repeating: **The scientific understanding of radicals has not yet led to any therapeutic application.** In fact, I can not think of one major medical breakthrough based exclusively on the free radical theory.

For many years, scavenging radicals with antioxidants was considered to be the most promising therapeutic approach, but clinical trials based on this principle have yielded mostly negative results. (Wingler, Schmidt, 2009).

In the light of my new model of disease causation and coexistence, the paradoxical controversy over oxidation is resolved. (my model is described in: *UTOPIA; The Medical and Scientific Significance of Oxygen Metabolism; Reactive Oxygen Species Insufficiency (ROSI) as the Basis for Disease Allowance and Coexistence: Extraordinary*

Support for an Extraordinary Theory; "The Oxypocalypse" or The war that never was"; *Death in Small Doses?; and Antioxidant Overkill).*

As with cancer, in cardiovascular disease, one can "cherry pick" some studies which suggest that antioxidants are good, bad or indifferent (without any effect at all). That is because there is such a wide spectrum of results from positive to negative to ineffective. However, either one has to dismiss all of the research (pro, con and neutral) or one has to look for a valid impression from the overall data.

There is certainly **a cautionary danger** in this but it is our only viable option at this point in the long history of our medical/scientific learning curve. Thus, I have followed the preponderance of the overall data in arriving at my conclusions. It stands the best chance of being right over the long haul.

Personal introductory comments: "Radical Planet"

Our environment is effectively saturated with electronically modified oxygen derivatives (EMODs). **We live on a "radical planet."**

Singlet oxygen, a name given to several higher energy species of molecular oxygen in which all the electron spins are paired, is much more reactive towards common organic molecules. In nature, singlet oxygen is commonly formed from water during photosynthesis, using the energy of sunlight. It is also produced by the immune system as a source of active oxygen.

The air and the water are fundamentally filled with hydrogen peroxide, superoxide anion, the hydroxyl radical and singlet oxygen. **Yet, the birds and the bees have not fallen from the sky, the aquatic dwellers are not floating belly-up and the surface occupiers are upright and flourishing.**

The dreaded **"oxypocalypse"** has not materialized as predicted by the free radical theorists. These free radical preachers of doom and gloom have invalidated their own brainwashed theory by its inherent lack of predictability and its inconsistencies.

Immune systems of higher organisms have long made use of reactive forms of oxygen which they produce. **Not only do antibodies catalyze production of peroxide from oxygen, it is now known that immune cells produce peroxide, superoxide, and singlet oxygen in the course of an immune response.** Recently, singlet oxygen has been found to be a source of biologically-produced ozone: this reaction proceeds through an unusual compound dihydrogen trioxide, also known as trioxidant, (HOOOH) which is an antibody-catalyzed product of singlet oxygen and water. This compound in turn disproportionates to ozone and peroxide, providing two powerful antibacterials.

I am convinced that a state of health is due to the constant warding off of disease. This is not particularly a new general concept but my proposal for the salutary role of EMODs is uniquely new. These diseases are frequently the result of bacteria, viruses, fungi, parasites and neoplasia (cancer development). Shielding us from disease is, in part, accomplished by the "continuously operational intrinsic oxidative defensive system," and that is conceptually unique.

I have racked my brain to find the most egregious examples for making my case that EMODs are beneficial essentials and are, in fact, of low toxicity. On the one hand, patients with chronic granulomatous disease (CGD) can not produce superoxide anions and they are subject to repeated infections and tumors called granulomas. These CGD conditions ultimately culminate in their early deaths. Further, Russian studies have shown that rats and mice raised in a superoxide-free atmosphere will die in 2-3 weeks. Additionally, knock out mice, which lack the gene which makes superoxide dismutase (SOD), quickly die. Please remember that SOD functions to produce H_2O_2 from superoxide. This fact makes SOD a prooxidant; not an antioxidant. Swiss acatalasemics, who can not produce catalase to break down H_2O_2, live essentially normal lives. Thus, I ask, "How toxic is H_2O_2?"

Myeloperoxidase (MPO) serves an unexpected, protective function in atherosclerosis in a hypercholesterolemic murine model and it generates hypochlorous acid (HOCl). *The free radical theory states that EMODs are causal for atherosclerosis (heart disease) but decreased levels of superoxide do not prevent atherosclerosis. Additionally,* **individuals with total MPO** deficiency show a high incidence of malignant tumors. These facts are strong arguments and support for my Unified theory and they serve as powerful arguments against the free radical theory.

Also, patients with glutathione peroxidase I deficiency live basically normal lives. Again, illustrating the low toxicity of EMODs.

Adipocytes of obese patients exhibit inflammation and hypoxia and have limited capability to generate EMODs. Obese patients are subject to increased risk of infections, delayed wound healing, diabetes, cancer and cataract formation. Obviously, I believe that these circumstances are directly related to decreased EMOD generation and to the development of a condition that I call **"Howes' EMOD insufficiency syndrome."** [The ROSI (reactive oxygen species insufficiency) syndrome of Howes].

Immunosuppressed patients (EMOD insufficiency patients) are subject to infections and cancer. In 2001, 62,000 people in the United States died of influenza or pneumonia. And each year, around 215,000 people in the United States die from severe sepsis, which is more than die from breast, colorectal, pancreatic, and prostate cancer combined. Tuberculosis, once considered under control, now kills 1.7 million every year. At the same time, new infectious diseases are emerging around the globe in such forms as bird flu and severe acute respiratory syndrome (SARS). I believe that these patients have an "endogenous EMOD insufficiency state." (Reactive Oxygen Species Insufficiency syndrome, **The ROSI syndrome of Howes**).

Bolstering their oxidative capacity could provide pathogen protection and disease prevention.

We now know that all antibody immune reactions involve the participation of EMODs, such as H_2O_2, hypochlorous acid, ozone and singlet oxygen. Prooxidant protection is crucial in combating bacterial, fungal, viral, and protozoan pathogens. HIV/AIDS patients suffer from repeated infections and Kaposi's sarcoma. These patients have a lacking ability to generate EMODs. Please remember that diabetes and arthritis are considered to be associated with immunosuppression by many authors and I believe that they are also related to an EMOD insufficiency.

There is no doubt that oxidation represents our first line of defense against pathogens and neoplasia. We know that the proper healing of wounds requires the participation of EMOD generating enzymes and without adequate collagen synthesis, normal healing can not occur. This is an obvious example of oxidative self healing.

On the other hand, hyperbilirubinemic babies treated with phototherapy, which specifically generates excited singlet oxygen, are not only cured of their jaundice but they live normal lives and attain normal life spans. These babies have been exposed to EMODs at one of the most vulnerable times of their lives (they have low antioxidant enzyme levels, their diet does not contain many of the low molecular weight antioxidants and colostrum is high in hydrogen peroxide), yet, they suffer no ill effects of these high doses of singlet oxygen. **In fact, these babies are suffering from a build up of the antioxidant, bilirubin, and are cured by the generation of an EMOD, singlet oxygen.**

I can not find an example of increased risks for common diseases, erroneously attributed to EMODs, following phototherapy (intentional generation of reactive oxygen species).

Free radical theorists predicted that combining iron and peroxide would produce the deleterious and possibly mutagenic hydroxyl radical, via the Fenton reaction, resulting in damaging carcinogenesis because of uncontrolled reactions of the hydroxyl radical with proteins and DNA.

Countless patients (millions) have irrigated, flushed, washed, and debrided wounds with 3% H_2O_2 for decades and by doing so have directly combined H_2O_2 with hemoglobin-iron at the injury or bleeding site. According to the free radical theory, this combination of H_2O_2 and iron should predictably produce the mutagenic and damaging hydroxyl radical but I can not find even one example of tumors or cancers at these sites in the literature. In fact, all I can find are examples of H_2O_2 aiding in the killing of pathogens, increasing local oxygen levels and augmenting wound healing.

Exercise has proven to be of great overall benefit to generalized health and to serve as an adjunct in the treatment of conditions considered to be caused by high levels of EMODs, such as diabetes, cancer, atherosclerosis, obesity and arthritis. Unquestionably, exercise always results in generation of high levels of EMODs and they are subsequently associated with salutary effects, reduction of diseases and their comorbidity and not related to harmful sequelae.

In my sixth book (*Diabetes and Oxygen Free Radical Sophistry,*), I was only going to discuss and review diabetes but it readily became apparent that I would have to include discussions of obesity, hypertension and atherosclerosis as well, since they are intimately linked to the diabetic condition. Additionally, **obesity has been linked to chronic diseases, such as type 2 diabetes, cardiovascular disease, hypertension and stroke, and some forms of cancer.**

Further, I wished to present an overview of my electronically modified oxygen derivative deficiency (**EMOD insufficiency) syndrome, which includes cancer,** atherosclerosis, strokes, obesity, diabetes, arthritis, hypertension, premature aging and cataracts. Many of these diseases serve as risk factors for others in this group.

Having a risk factor for a disease makes the chances of getting that disease higher but does not always lead to development of the disease. Also, the absence of any risk factors or having a protective factor does not necessarily guard you against getting the disease. There are other cases where one disease is associated with an increased risk of having another.

Major trials do not prove the value of antioxidant vitamins. In fact, hundreds have failed. They show that many of the so called antioxidant benefits have been overstated and that there may be many serious adverse effects associated with their use. Currently, clinical trial results are our best way to assess the risks and benefits of antioxidant supplements. However, although occasional positive responses have been reported with these agents, hundreds of reports have shown no benefit. Yet, there are widespread disparities in the literature.

My work is not going to be just a step forward, it's going to be a potential revolution. Once we have identified the mechanism for disease causation, steps can be logically taken for control, prevention or cure of some disease entities, possibly cancer, heart disease, AIDS and malaria.

Ninety nine percent of today's medical and scientific papers assume or accept the validity of the free radical theory and the concept of so-called oxidative stress. The literature is filled with erroneous prejudice towards EMODs. Investigators design their studies to validate the erroneous Free Radi-Crap theory and when their results fail to do so, they seriously question their very own experiments.

Medical Headlines, Spurious Associations and Junk Science

It is estimated that there are currently 25 thousand medical/scientific journals turning out over one million publications annually.

It is also estimated that 50% of these papers have reached the wrong conclusions.

Personally, I feel that the percentage of erroneous conclusions is higher than their estimate. I keep one computer file on "spurious (meaning not genuine, false, fake, etc.) associations" for medical/scientific papers. Large studies lend themselves to misinterpretation and misrepresentation of underlying facts.

Slick advertisers capitalize on these ludicrous false associations. So-called observational or epidemiological studies have especially been prone to drawing false conclusions, i.e. elderly people have gray hair; so, gray hair causes aging.

This false conclusion is wrong and only shows an "association" of graying of the hair and aging. Association is not causation. Strange things happen when statistical analysis is applied to medical science.

Some "headline" examples of recent spurious associations in the medical literature are as follows: "Large thighs may protect the heart," "Short legs linked to liver disease," "Short limbs linked with higher risk of memory loss," "Women eating one quarter grapefruit a day had 30% higher risk of breast cancer," "Rainfall autism theory suggested," "Autumn babies at greater risk of asthma," "Watching TV increases risk of autism," "Cell phones can affect sperm quality," "Hairspray linked to birth defects," and "Too much TV linked to higher asthma risk."

We must carefully evaluate all studies, apply good old common sense (in addition to scientific scrutiny) and avoid acceptance of unusual conclusions with blind faith or religious fervor.

Studies that report a link between some new risk factor and disease are everywhere and frequently mean little or nothing. Do not take the hook, remain somewhat skeptical and await actual proof, before adopting life style changes or swallowing the latest "magic pill."

Be wary of strange medical claims. We must remain enthusiastic concerning medical science but must also be dedicated to truthful reporting. It is ironic that accepting nonsense medical "headlines" may be your greatest medical risk factor for your overall well being.

Be especially wary of medical claims by Dr. Mehmet Oz. This Oprah-wanna-be spews more untruths than the U.S. Congress.

Benjamin Franklin had stated in the Declaration of Independence, **"We hold these truths to be self evident."** Franklin had borrowed this term from Newton. Scientists, including Einstein, had tried to describe natural phenomenon with theories of unification. I have done similarly with the biological systems which utilize oxygen metabolism and I believe that I have presented facts regarding oxygen metabolism which are self evident, with respect to its essentiality and its low toxicity, even though this contradicts many in vitro experiments. The magic occurs in the living/breathing cell. In vitro experiments are filled with "dead artifacts" conducted in Pyrex glass coffins.

My work is bolstered by the application of **Occam's razor or the rule of parsimony,** in that the simplest explanation is usually the right answer. The most basic aspect of disease manifestation is alterations in oxygen and EMOD levels. Oxygen-related metabolism is a key factor in "allowing" disease causation, and in maintaining homeostasis, prooxidant protection and oxidative self healing. It is crucial in the maintenance of a continually operational intrinsic oxidative defensive system for protection against pathogens, heart disease and cancer.

I have attempted to keep abstracts in a recognizable form and thus have not labeled them as such. Also, I have tried my very best to be certain to reference all materials, which are extensive and which are cited in my book.

If one were to take the literature on oxygen free radicals (EMODs) in its entirety, one would probably be led to discount all theories since results are spread all over the place and filled with inconsistencies. In other words, when there exists diametrically opposed data, which is the correct data? Or, can it be that both are correct? Or, is it such that both are wrong? Should one cherry-pick the data?

The widely varying and confusing risk measurements from different studies raises a question as to a proper risk value for CVD. It is said that there are over 100 risk factors for heart disease. Knowledge about the key mechanisms that cause a disease is a usual requirement for designing methods to reduce or eliminate its risk.

It has been said that one must use caution in recommending antioxidant supplements to people with heart disease, cancer or diabetes. One basis for this caution is that, under certain circumstances, vitamin E or C can actually act as a prooxidant.

Actually, nearly all antioxidants can have prooxidant activity, usually to a lesser extent than the original antioxidant. Also, vitamin C shares several cellular transport mechanisms with glucose, and it can increase the rate of absorption of iron, which is a prooxidant. However, because of years of study, I do not believe that this prooxidant activity is as harmful as is their antioxidant activity, especially in situations in which there is an antioxidant overload. Please read my book entitled, *Antioxidant Overkill.*

A lack of oxygenation leads to a lack of oxidation by EMODs, which leads to or "allows" for disease manifestation. Ground state oxygen lacks the reactivity necessary to participate in the complex biochemical reactions required to maintain homeostasis, to protect us against pathogens and to sustain our health. Intermediate EMODs are sufficiently reactive to protect and to heal us. However, **an antioxidant surfeit or electron over abundance reduces oxygen and its EMODs to non-reactive water.**

Additionally, each EMOD species must be considered separately due to differences in reaction characteristics and chemical qualities. We can no longer carelessly and incorrectly lump them under one erroneous and misleading heading, such as reactive oxygen species.

The use of the term "oxidative stress" is misleading and overlooks the fact that oxygen species are in a state of constant change (flux) in the organelles, the cell itself, the tissue and the entire aerobic organism. Our redox status is a constantly changing and dynamic system. There is an electron flow throughout all aerobic organisms and this flow must be maintained. Even visionary, Albert Szent Gyorgi, realized that, "without electron and proton flow, we are dead."

As I said in my book entitled, *Medical and Scientific Significance of Oxygen Free Radical Metabolism,* "The primary process which stands between us and constant or perpetual infections or manifestations of neoplasia, is our ability to generate oxidative events in the form of EMODs and electron and proton movement, which form a major part of our "intrinsic, continually operational, oxidative, defensive system." (Howes, 2005)

Cyclic neutropenia, chronic granulomatous disease and spontaneous regression of cancer illustrate my point. Neutrophils produce pathogen-protective EMODs. It appears that the key players, among others, in the immune system, in preventing infections and cancer, are antibodies, macrophages, lymphocytes, neutrophils, T-cells and Interleukin-2. All of these can and do generate or stimulate EMOD production. Antibodies can generate hydrogen peroxide (H_2O_2) from singlet molecular oxygen ($^1O_2{}^*$). Antibodies produce up to 500 mole equivalents of H_2O_2 from $^1O_2{}^*$, without a reduction in rate. There is an enormous potential for H_2O_2 production by antibodies. **I believe that this inter-relationship between $^1O_2^*$, H_2O_2 and O_3 will prove to have great significance in the generation of a DOA (deadly oxidative assault) and prooxidant protection towards cancer and disease.**

Oxygen plays a pivotal role in the maintenance of life for all eukaryotes, with the exception of strict anaerobes. Eukaryotes have developed mechanisms to sense and respond to decreased oxygen levels and to deal with EMODs safely.

All living aerobic organisms have adaptive mechanisms to maintain oxygen homeostasis.

Antioxidant vitamins demonstrate how a therapy that is reportedly safe, because it allegedly has no biochemical effect, can do damage. If antioxidants had significant biochemical effects, as claimed, they should be classified as drugs. People say antioxidant vitamin ingestion cannot do any harm but when it is being promoted for cancer, heart disease and stroke cures, then there is a serious problem. Making false claims about treating colds (or the sniffles) is one thing but it is quite another to make false claims about the reversal of heart disease, aging or curing cancer.

With collision analysis, we struggle to determine
the inner working quantum characteristics of the atom
and its subatomic clan.
Fission, fusion and scatter have yielded scant knowledge
of their non-Newtonian world.
Yet, even the slightest of these particles
knows all of the inherent quantum laws and
follows them explicitly.
They have demonstrated this to us in the box-car letters,
spelled out on the periodic table.
Their distinctive behavior demonstrates
their inherently distinctive knowledge.
They are the site of the cognitive atomic and
molecular thinking matrix, which dictates
the habits of the world,
and which envelops all.
R. M. Howes, M.D., Ph.D.
11/15/06

My opinion on EMODs and antioxidant vitamins in a nut shell

"You have enemies? Good. That means you've stood up for something, some-
time in your life."
 -Winston Churchill

For decades, reports have praised the benefits of the antioxidant vitamins and
assailed the role of EMODs. Investigators and marketers attempted to stack up
enough "anecdotal maybes" that they hoped to create the illusion of a scientific
definite but recent randomized controlled trials have blown these charlatans
out of the waters of scientific truth. Yet, they continue to swim in the shallows
of biochemical ignorance and the dangerous currents of denial.

In 2007, **Dr. Michael Sporn, past Head of the National Cancer Institute
Chemoprevention Laboratory and current professor of pharmacology and
toxicology at Dartmouth Medical School and Eminent Scholar, NCI's Center
for Cancer Research, said that, "The use of dietary substances, like the antioxidant vitamins C and E, has been pretty much a colossal failure for protection against almost any kind of human disease."**

Epiphanies of 11-05-07

**During the evening of 11-05-07, I had two epiphanies: 1) all things age
including subatomic particles. We call it "decay" instead of aging in this
instance. 2) antioxidant vitamins can be thought of as "precursors to oxidants." They could be considered harmful because they wait around to dump
electrons on oxidants and thus, negate or nullify the beneficial effects of
oxidants. It all depends on how one looks at it. As with so many things, it is
a matter of perspective.**

However, I say that the antioxidant vitamins A and E, and to a lesser extent
vitamin C, have performed their functions beautifully (which is not the prevention of cancer, heart disease or strokes), which is their role in assisting oxidants
as electron donors and to **serve as precursors** to more oxidants, which they ultimately also become once they lose an electron. The free radical theory (FRT)
has been an uber-colossal failure. I can find no diseases, other than routine
vitamin deficiencies, which are prevented or reversed by the administration of
the antioxidant vitamins. Actually, risk for common diseases are increased and
an early demise is associated with their use.

The FRT was based on poor and inappropriately applied radiation science and a preponderance of subsequent scientific data has now invalidated the free radical theory. Please read both of my companion books, i.e., *Death In Small Doses?* and *Antioxidant Overkill*. **Currently, there is abundant significant scientific data which nullifies the FRT.** (Howes, 2010)

Yet, the FRT has been so ingrained into current medico-scientific thinking that it continues to bias countless studies and the consequent analysis and interpretation of data. Investigators are reportedly "disappointed" in their results, when these antioxidant vitamins fail to perform as predicted by the FRT and rarely question the flawed theory upon which their predictions were based. Rather than question the free radical theory, they prefer to question their own data. Balanced nutrition **and exercise, not antioxidant supplements, should be emphasized for overall health.**

CHAPTER SEVEN

"Life's tough......it's even tougher if you're stupid.."
- John Wayne

Coexisting or clustering of diseases and the Howes EMOD insufficiency syndrome (The ROSI Syndrome of Howes)

Throughout my many years of research on oxygen metabolism, I have been impressed with the clustering of certain diseases , such as cancer, diabetes, atherosclerosis (heart disease), arthritis, cataracts, obesity, HIV/AIDS, immunosuppression and Alzheimer's disease. The presence of only one of these diseases tends to increase the risk for another of this group. Thus, the obvious question is, "Why?" Clues to this query are hidden throughout the vast vista of the scientific literature, including genetics.

A risk factor is anything that increases a person's chance of getting a disease. Some risk factors can be changed and others cannot. For example, risk factors for cancer can include a person's age, sex, and family medical history. Others are linked to cancer-causing factors in the environment. Still others are related to lifestyle choices such as tobacco and alcohol use, diet, and sun exposure.

Having a risk factor for a disease means that a person is more likely to develop the disease at some point in their lives. However, having one or more risk factors does not necessarily mean that a person will get the disease. Some people with one or more risk factors never develop the disease, while other people who do develop the disease have no apparent risk factors.

Even when a person who has a risk factor is diagnosed with, for instance, cancer and heart disease, there is no way to prove that the risk factor actually caused the cancer or the CVD.

Association is not tantamount to causation.

I have been impressed that two of the most influential factors for heart disease appear to be depression (along with anxiety and stress), which significantly worsens the condition, and ingestion of nuts, which lowers heart disease risks, even though they are high in omega-6 fatty acids.

Patients taking long term cortisone tend to develop skin cancer and lymphomas, high blood glucose (diabetes), cardiovascular disease, thin skin, repeated infections, osteoporosis, impaired immune system, siphoning of fat from the arms and legs and depositing of it in the face and trunk, weakened muscles, cataracts and poor wound healing. **My studies lead me to believe that most of these conditions are due to an EMOD insufficiency. The fact that long term ingestion of steroids causes the development of these conditions speaks volumes about their inter-relationships.**

Investigators have recently demonstrated that **reactive oxygen species (ROS, EMODs) generation by polymorphonuclear leukocytes (PMNL) and mononuclear cells (MNC) is inhibited following the intravenous administration of hydrocortisone.** This is associated with a parallel decrease in intranuclear NFκB, known to modulate inflammatory responses including ROS generation. They have also shown that the plasma levels of interleukin-10 (IL-10), an anti-inflammatory and immunosuppressive cytokine produced by TH2 cells, are also increased after hydrocortisone administration. (Dandona et al, 2001) (Paresh Dandona et al. Acute suppressive effect of hydrocortisone on p47[phox] subunit of nicotinamide adenine dinucleotide phosphate oxidase. Metabolism. Volume 50, Issue 5, May 2001, Pages 548-552).

> *We knew that HIV infection or AIDS weakens the immune system*
> *and makes people at least 800 times more likely to have*
> *their latent TB infection activated. It wasn't realized until later*
> *that the reverse is also true: Active tuberculosis further suppresses*
> *the immune system of AIDS patients; curing tuberculosis actually*
> *improves the immune system.*
> Lee B. Reichman,

Timebomb: The Global Epidemic of
Multi-Drug-Resistant Tuberculosis,
2002, New York: McGraw Hill

I believe that just as one disease lowers the immune system and predisposes to another disease, that lowering of the EMOD level also predisposes to the occurrence of another disease (disease coexistence). They can have a cumulative EMOD lowering effect and produce the clustering I have discussed, which is secondary to an overall EMOD insufficiency.

Supplements and Pills: What Will Americans Swallow?

When it comes to advertisements and supplement pills, Americans will pay premium prices to swallow darned near anything.

Estimates vary but we spend up to a whopping $27 billion annually on supplements that have not been tested for safety, effectiveness or quality. With over 40,000 products on the market, who can possibly keep an eye on this gargantuan market?

The Food and Drug Administration (FDA) can not regulate our medicines properly, let alone the additional load of the supplement industry. Dietary supplements, antioxidants, vitamins and neutraceuticals are gobbled up faster than a sizzling T-bone by a starved dog.

We buy fish oil that doesn't even come from fish, lead-laden ginkgo pills, vitamin laced water, dressed up junk food and arsenic tainted herbals at premium prices. We do this because we have been misled to believe that these products really are "ancient Chinese discoveries," "anti-aging pills," "instant weight loss medicines" or "miracle cures" that orthodox medicine wants to hide from us.

Actually, most of the scientific studies that have been done on many of the antioxidants and vitamins have shown that they totally lack effectiveness and that they are potentially harmful. The only place that they actually do some good is in folks with known vitamin deficiencies.

Additionally, with today's foods being "fortified" with antioxidants and vitamins, and with consumers taking literally tons of these supplements, experts are warning about the possibility of over dosing on many of these products.

According to a 2002 report in the New England Journal of Medicine, "Tens of thousands of supplement-related health problems are handled by U.S. poison control centers each year." Not until 2008 were supplement makers required to report problems to the FDA, and then it was only for serious problems. The FDA estimates that there are over 50,000 safety problems yearly related to supplement use.

The Medicated States of America

Relentless advertising by the uber rich pharmaceutical industry has officially made the United States the pill-popping, drug-guzzling champion of the world.

Experts say that one-third of U.S. adults take five or more prescription medicines or supplements. It should be no surprise that some **18 million people end up in hospital emergency rooms each year because of medication errors.** Tragically, **over 106,000 annual deaths are attributed to adverse drug reactions.**

Studies by Medco Health Solutions Inc., which manages prescription benefits, found that for the first time, **51 percent of American children and adults were taking one or more prescription drugs for chronic health conditions.**

Commonly prescribed drugs for chronic diseases are those which treat high blood pressure and high cholesterol. Pain medicines and antidepressants are running a close second. Antidepressant use has jumped among teens and working-age women. The biggest jump in use of chronic medications was in the 20- to 44-year-old age group, where drugs are used to treat depression, diabetes, asthma, attention-deficit disorder and seizures.

The proportion of Americans on chronic medications will grow. In fact, drug companies have cut back on research on medicines to treat acute conditions, such as infections, because these medicines are only prescribed for short intervals of about a week; whereas, drugs for chronic conditions require a lifetime reliance on these much more profitable drugs.

Medication use for chronic problems was seen in 75% of people 65 or older and nearly 66% of women 20 and older. Some patients were found to take up to 20 medications a day, which can be a pill-popping nightmare.

There is good news and bad news. The good news is that, overall, we are living longer than ever before. The bad news is that we appear to be getting fatter, lazier and more dependent upon "quick fixes promised by medications and supplements" and less reliant upon the will power to exercise, watch our weight and eat a healthy, nutritious diet.

The Powerful Placebo Effect

In both traditional and alternative medicine, the placebo effect looms large as long as patients "believe" in the potion, healer or procedure. In a recent study of a drug to relieve the symptoms of lupus, about a third felt better when they received the dummy pills instead of the actual drug.

Basically, that means that placebo treatments can (and do) have significant desirable medicinal effects, especially if you believe in it. This is particularly true with pain, since it is subjective.

Estimates are that the placebo effect is responsible for about one third of the benefits of any treatment. Because I am a physician and a scientist, this is hard to accept but "the results are what they are." The placebo effect began being studied in 1955 by H.K. Beecher with his ground breaking work reporting "The Powerful Placebo."

We must acknowledge the fact that the human mind can influence our health in a major way, both good and bad. We should also admit that the body can manifest an almost miraculous ability for "self cure." Placebo can be a doctor's best ally. Keep positive thoughts, never give up and always push forward. As I once advised a long termed depressed patient, "You can change everything by simply changing your attitude."

The Free Radi-Crap Theory (FRT)
The only justifiable reason
for the existence of the free radical theory,
is to make tarot card reading
appear to be respectable.
R.M. Howes M.D., Ph.D.
3/22/06

FRT is a meretricious (plausible but false) theory.

In 1956, Dr. Denham Harman proposed the free radical theory, whereby oxygen free radicals supposedly were the cause for over 100 human diseases including cancer, heart disease and aging. (Harman, 1956).

Free radicals are chemicals which have unpaired outer orbital electrons and were thought to have damaging reactivity with biological molecules such as lipids, proteins and nucleic acids. In vitro laboratory animal studies and epidemiologic observations seemed to support the free radical theory. **Thereafter, electronically modified oxygen derivatives (EMODs) were progressively demonized in the scientific literature and later free radicals were widely debased in the lay publications.**

The free radical theory of aging, elaborated and first investigated mainly by Harman and later by many others, **suggests that oxygen free radicals are harmful byproducts of aerobic life and as such represent the basic cause of aging and numerous diseases** (Harman, 1957) (Harman, 1961) (Harman, 1981) (Harman, 1988) (Harman, 1992) (Harman, 1994).

Antioxidants were touted as the savior from the alleged damaging effects of EMODs and were quickly called to the rescue. Antioxidants are chemicals which were believed to nullify, scavenge or eliminate free radicals and were predicted to be the answer to "free radical caused diseases" in man. Scientists readily assumed three things: 1) that the free radical theory was correct, 2) that oxygen free radicals were deleterious and 3) that antioxidants would successfully counteract the damaging effects of oxygen free radicals.

They were wrong on all three counts.

In vitro studies have shown that cells can be damaged by reactions with free radicals. Thus, it was assumed that living/breathing cells would respond in a similar fashion and that free radicals were the causative factor for over 100 pathophysiologies, including cancer, cardiovascular disease and aging. **Dr. Denham Harman had planted the seed of confusion which led to the growth of a sprawling tree of erroneous free radical hypotheses, over shadowing the real truth in regards to oxygen free radicals and human disease causation.**

Tens of thousands of scientific papers have been published on this subject and most of those published in the later half of the 20th century were interpreted as being supportive of the free radical theory, until the 1990s. Yet, the literature was filled with "paradoxes" and inconsistencies. Dietary antioxidant supplements were the rage. However, large, randomized, double blind, controlled studies subsequent to this have not only demonstrated that antioxidants are frequently ineffective in the prevention of the alleged "free radical caused diseases" but that they were also the source of potential harm or death.

When confronted with non-supportive evidence, the medico-scientific establishment did what any purveyor of profitable misinformation would do, i.e., they either ignore it or call it a paradox and move on. Interestingly, they simultaneously seek out supportive evidence, no matter how flimsy, and then embark on an aggressive propaganda campaign to 'indoctrinate' as many people as possible to this allegedly supportive evidence. The end result is that the general public receives a highly distorted version of events that, while far from the truth, is nonetheless far more palatable to the reigning orthodoxy. Thus, all is well in the kingdom. The last thing they want is controversy and questioning of the reigning dogma. So it has been with the free radical theory for the last fifty years.

Heart disease predetermined by oxygen levels in the womb

The amount of oxygen available to a baby in the womb can affect their susceptibility to developing particular diseases later in life. Research presented at the annual Society for Endocrinology BES meeting in Harrogate shows that your risk of developing cardiovascular disease can be predetermined before birth, not only by your genes, but also by their interaction with the quality of the environment you experience in the womb.

Researchers at the University of Cambridge, led by Dr Dino Giussani, examined the role that **oxygen availability** in the womb plays in programming your susceptibility to different diseases. His group found that **babies that don't receive enough oxygen in the womb (e.g. due to pre-eclampsia or placental insufficiency) are more likely to suffer from cardiovascular disease when they are adult.**

A reduction of oxygen levels in the womb can lead to reduced growth rates in the baby and to changes in the way that their cardiovascular, metabolic and endocrine systems develop. Combined, these alterations to the development of key systems in the body can leave the baby more prone to developing cardiovascular disease later in life. I believe that it is obvious that less oxygen availability results in an EMOD insufficiency and to an increased risk for developing clustering of diseases, such as seen with my ROSI syndrome.

Dr Giussani's research also indicates methods by which we can potentially combat this problem. The detrimental effects of low oxygen levels on the development of the unborn's cardiovascular system appear to be due to the generation of oxidative stress.

I disagree, due to the many studies showing that hypoxia does not result in an increase in EMOD production. I can argue on the basis of the law of mass action or the rules of stochiometry that lower levels of EMODs are produced when the oxygen substrate is present in rate limiting amounts.

Treatment with antioxidants in animal pregnancies complicated by low oxygenation can "allegedly" reverse these effects on the developing cardiovascular system and this could form the basis for new therapeutic techniques to prevent the early origin of heart disease in complicated human pregnancy.

Cardiovascular disease is the most common cause of death in the UK, accounting for 4 in every 10 deaths. Almost 2.6 million people are affected by heart and circulatory conditions in the UK, with someone having a heart attack every 2 seconds.

Scientist Dr Dino Giussani said: "We have known for a while that changes in maternal nutrition can affect fetal development and influence disease susceptibility later in life, but relatively little work has investigated how low oxygen levels in the womb may affect infant development. Our research shows that changes to the amount of oxygen available in the womb can have a profound influence on the development of the fetus in both the short and long- term, and trigger an early origin of heart disease.

Interestingly and allegedly, Giussani believes the adverse effects on the developing heart and circulation of poor fetal oxygenation are due to oxidative stress. This gives us the opportunity to combat prenatal origins of heart disease by fetal exposure to antioxidant therapy. This may halt the development of heart disease at its very origin, bringing preventative medicine back into the womb." To me, it would seem more logical to merely increase the oxygen supply to normal levels for the developing fetus or embryo.

The paper was presented at the Society for Endocrinology BES meeting on April 8, 2008. This work was funded by the British Heart Foundation, The Royal Society, The Lister Institute for Preventive Medicine, the BBSRC and the Isaac Newton Trust.

The body's susceptibility to so called oxidant damage is thought to depend on the **balance** between the extent of prooxidant levels and the antioxidant levels of body tissues. **Most antioxidants have a large number of alternating double bonds which can act as electron traps.** In some cases, **this quenching reaction can lead to increased oxidation.**

This occurs when a polyunsaturated fat (such as omega-3) neutralizes an oxygen radical but becomes a fatty acid radical which then attacks another lipid leading to a chain reaction. **Thus, there is no distinct division between "good antioxidants" and "bad oxidants." One can and does become the other. Once an antioxidant gives its electron to an oxidant, that antioxidant immediately becomes a radical oxidant itself. Please remember that this is not the case for antioxidant enzymes.**

Other antioxidants can also act as prooxidants after quenching an oxygen radical. On balance, a number of studies have shown that various antioxidants act as a cooperative system of antioxidant defense **but all antioxidants may have prooxidant activity or potential. Please remember this point.**

Here is how I see it:

There is no doubt that antioxidants such as vitamins A, C and E have antioxidant properties and activity.

There is also no doubt that reliable studies have shown that these antioxidants can cause increased risks for heart attacks, congestive heart failure, strokes and overall mortality.

There is also no doubt that oxidants (EMODs) are our first line of defense against infections and neoplasia.

While there remains some uncertainty about the long term effects of antioxidant supplementation there is little evidence that the practice of dietary supplementation may be beneficial, and it has the potential to be harmful.

The free radical theory has prejudiced countless studies and clouded interpretation of data ever since it was introduced. It has progressed to the point of absurdity, such that **if an investigators' results are not in agreement with the free radical theory, that investigator considers his results to be a paradox or that his study was flawed.** Investigators are reluctant to offer explanations which go against the dogma of the erroneous free radical theory.

It has swayed scientific opinion such that bias (which I italicized below) is now part of the definition of supposedly scientific terms as follows:

Antioxidant -An enzyme or other organic molecule that can counteract the *damaging effects of oxygen in tissues*

Free Radical -An atom or a molecule with an unpaired electron, *highly reactive* with nearby molecules. Free radical damage may be countered with antioxidants

Oxidative *Stress* -A state in which the effects of prooxidants exceed the ability of antioxidant systems to neutralize them

Reactive oxygen species (ROS, some EMODs) - *Highly reactive chemicals, containing oxygen, that react easily with other molecules resulting in potentially damaging modifications*

All of these terms indicate that oxygen free radicals are only capable of harmful effects and that antioxidants are wonderfully helpful agents within our cells. **This is basically wrong and is another example of nonscience/nonsense.**

We have been told that dietary antioxidant vitamins and antioxidants obtained from dietary fruits and vegetables would be the godsend in eliminating the deleterious oxygen free radicals and consequently, the occurrence of the host of disease which they allegedly caused. **That has not proven to be the case.**

> "You are being radically misled
> by antioxidant vitamin fraudsters."
> Someone is trying to radically mislead you
> concerning antioxidant vitamins and
> antioxidant supplements,
> such that you will make
> a radical mistake."
> R.M. Howes M.D., Ph.D.
> 3/22/06

Reactions involving H_2O_2 are not subject to inhibition by classic antioxidants such as vitamin E.

The introduction of lipid-soluble antioxidants will limit lipid peroxidation but will have no effect on $2e$-oxidants and thus no effect on protein modification by $ONOO^-$, cell signaling by H_2O_2, or HOCl-mediated oxidation reactions.

Conversely, species that scavenge H_2O_2 will have a profound effect on HOCl-mediated oxidation but may also wipe out H_2O_2-mediated signaling,

A high vitamin C intake from supplements is associated with an increased risk of cardiovascular disease mortality in postmenopausal women with diabetes. (Lee et al, 2004).

Similarly, the clinical trials based on **high dose of dietary vitamin C supplement are not supportive**, although epidemiologic and observational studies based on food intake provide evidence for a strong protective role of vitamin C against **cancer**.

Paradoxically, in the presence of Fe^{3+} or $Cu^{2+,}$ ascorbate can promote the generation of the same reactive oxygen species ($.OH$, $O_2^{.-}$, H_2O_2, and ferryl ion) it is known to destroy. (Stadtman, 1991).

On the basis of an increased number of modified DNA basis in lymphocytes, Podmore et al **claimed that dietary supplementation with vitamin C at 500 mg/d exerts prooxidant and mutagenic effects in humans.** (Podmore et al, 1998).

Vitamin C, when taken as a dietary supplement, does not appear to reduce mortality in patients with cardiovascular disease. It has been suggested, *for half a century,* that antioxidant nutrients, such as vitamin C, may play a role in reducing cardiovascular disease.

The **U.S. Preventive Services Task Force (USPSTF)** conducted a systematic review of the studies on **vitamin C** and found the evidence **inconclusive** because the studies were inadequate and conflicting and that there is insufficient evidence to recommend vitamin supplements for the prevention of cardiovascular disease. (USPSTF, 2003).

Five studies included **102,735 patients** taking various doses of **vitamin C but showed no effect on cardiovascular disease mortality.** (Morris, Carson, 2003).

The party line of the oxy-morons is that uncontrolled blood glucose can promote the production of unhealthy oxidation reactions and foster many diseases, including arteriosclerosis. Hence, they believed that supplementing the diet with antioxidants, such as **vitamin C,** would benefit diabetics. A study by Jacobs et al in the Nov. 2004 issue of American Journal of Clinical Nutrition, found that **such supplements may actually promote the clogging of arteries.** They evaluated cardiovascular disease in **1,923 post-menopausal women with diabetes,** part of the **Iowa Women's Health Study,** which collected data in 1986 about diets and vitamin C consumption in nearly **35,000 recruits.** The researchers found that **women with diabetes consuming at least 300 milligrams of vitamin C per day faced 2.3 times the risk of death from stroke and 2 times the risk of dying from coronary artery disease** as did diabetic women who took in less of the vitamin C.

The Institute of Medicine in the US reports there's a total lack of evidence to show large doses of antioxidants protect us from disease. In the case of vitamin C, doses of over 2000 milligrams can cause diarrhea, and **mega doses may even accelerate cancer growth and harden the arteries.** The University of Pennsylvania found large doses of vitamin C triggered the release of DNA-damaging chemicals in the body, which may lead to cancer.

The antioxidant effects of vitamin C are well established but **vitamin C may also function as a prooxidant.** (Roussel et al, 2005). **Interestingly, only the DHA (oxidant) form of vitamin C can cross the blood brain barrier.**

Vitamin C and goats

The recommended daily dose of vitamin C for humans is just one mg/kg, while goats, for example, produce the vitamin at a striking rate of 200 mg/ kg each day. Incidentally, I found that skin cancer is fairly common in goats. Ergo, vitamin C does not prevent skin cancer in goats. Also, goats are used as a study model for the development of plaque formation following dietary supplement of cholesterol. I believe that this fact alone should put to rest the notion that mega-doses of vitamin C will prevent cancer and heart disease.

"As researchers and clinicians,
our most important criterion should be
indisputable safety, and
antioxidant therapy currently
falls woefully short of this benchmark.
R.M. Howes M.D., Ph.D.
3/17/06

Experts say that perhaps antioxidants work when they are in food, but not when in pills. Some even think antioxidants may have been a red herring and that maybe people who eat vitamin-rich food generally take better care of themselves and that's why they have lower disease risks.

Watch out for statistical fabrication and fuzzy math.

CHAPTER EIGHT

Dr. Mehmet OoZe presents
his daily hour-long TV infomercial,
"Pimping The Supplements"
R.M. Howes M.D., Ph.D.
2/3/12

Patient use of dietary supplements: a clinician's perspective

The estimated prevalence of dietary-supplement use among US adults was 73% in 2002. Appropriate use of dietary supplements within the paradigm of evidence-based medicine may be a challenge for medical doctors and non-physician clinicians. Randomized, controlled, clinical trial data, which are considered the gold standard for evidence-based decision making, are lacking. Standardized guidelines for the use of dietary supplements are lacking, and dietary supplements can bear unsupported claims. OBJECTIVES: This article is intended to review clinically-relevant issues related to the widespread use of dietary supplements, with emphasis on regulatory oversight and safety. METHODS: Review articles and clinical trial articles published up until December 2007 were selected based on a search of the MEDLINE electronic database using PubMed. The Food and Drug Administration (FDA) Website was also used as a resource. We used the search terms dietary supplement(s), vitamin supplements, mineral supplements, and Dietary Supplement and Health Education Act. Articles discussing dietary supplements and their regulation, prevalence of use, prescription and nonprescription formulations, and/or adverse events were selected for review. Articles discussing one or more of these topics in adults were selected for inclusion. RESULTS: New FDA regulations require dietary-supplement manufacturers to evaluate the identity, purity, strength, and composition of their products. However, these regulations are not designed to demonstrate product efficacy and safety, and dietary-supplement manufacturers are not required to submit efficacy and safety data to the FDA prior to marketing. Product contamination and/or mislabeling may undermine the integrity of dietary-supplement formulations. CONCLUSIONS: The use of dietary supplements may be associated with adverse events. Although there are new regulatory requirements for dietary supplements, these products will not require FDA approval or submission of efficacy and safety data prior to marketing under the new regulation. A limitation to the literature used for this review is the lack of prospective, randomized clinical trials on the safety and efficacy of dietary supplements. Clinicians should be aware of all the dietary supplements that their patients consume, and help their patients make informed decisions appropriate to their medical care. (Sadovosky et al, 2008)

Therapeutic Uses

Many health claims for antioxidant supplements are based on the fact that they are strong antioxidants. However, in recent years, scientific confidence in the medical benefits of antioxidants has waned dramatically; study after gigantic study of antioxidants, such as vitamin E and beta carotene, have failed to find the hoped-for (promised) benefits.

Antioxidant use

Antioxidant supplements are sold in combination with other supplements. Because of the widespread use of antioxidant supplements by 10% to 30% of the adult population (80-160 million people) in North America and Europe, this is a serious public health issue and the potential for harm or increased mortality is highly significant.

It now appears that antioxidant vitamins may be agents of "death in small doses" and it seems likely that this implies an associated legal liability and a significant public health safety issue.

Antioxidants can block crucial EMOD functions, including sperm and ova function, apoptosis, the respiratory burst, protein translation, phagocytosis and detoxification. Excessive antioxidants could dangerously interfere with these protective functions, while temporary depletion of antioxidants can enhance anti-cancer effects of apoptosis.

I believe that EMODs are of low toxicity and are essential secondary cellular messengers. We must endeavor to maintain adequate levels of prooxidant protection from pathogens and neoplasia. Also, we must maintain adequate EMOD levels to sustain their crucial role as secondary messengers in components of reproduction. Without this, reproduction will not occur.

The lofty predictions of the discredited free radical theory, as regards the ability of antioxidants to prevent, nullify or reverse mankind's common diseases and aging have fallen woefully short. To the contrary, the antioxidant vitamins actually increase the risk of the diseases they were supposed to cure or prevent and they increase mortality.

At this point in time, randomized controlled trials have accumulated convincing data showing the ineffectiveness and dangers of common antioxidants, such as vitamins beta carotene, A, C and E. These same vitamins are promoted and marketed with near reckless abandon regarding consumer safety.

Because of the quantity and quality of the scientific data, there is now a legal and moral liability issue associated with their unrestrained use. We must make patient and consumer safety our number one priority.

In an August 2011 article entitled, *Is Cancer Beating Cardiovascular disease?*, **Clyde Yancy MD, chief of cardiology at Northwestern University, Chicago, IL, who serves on the FDA's Circulatory System Devices Committee, said, "We willingly accept and prescribe without hesitation chemotherapy agents that we recognize will put a patient at risk of developing heart failure, and I wouldn't advocate against that because those drugs, those Adriamycin-type compounds, are critical in the fight against certain types of cancers. *But if there is any cardiovascular drug for which there is even a hint that a contribution to malignancies might occur, it would be totally unacceptable to allow a drug on the market,* even if it had a clinical experience of being beneficial."**

I believe that this same degree of caution should exist for the overuse of antioxidants, which have been proven to increase the risk of disease and death.

Yet, when it comes to antioxidants, we allow them to be sold freely over the counter to an unsuspecting public. Not only do they increase the risk of cancer, but they significantly increase the risk of a host of other serious diseases, such as heart disease, strokes, diabetes, fractures, premature births, sperm damage, etc.

None of the entire group of dietary supplements are government tested for efficacy or safety. This must stop. The public has been conditioned to believe that anyone arguing for the testing of supplements is in kahoots with the pharmaceutical industry and that any regulation of these potentially harmful agents will significantly raise their cost of non-prescription supplements.

An increasing number of studies are finding that vitamin supplementation are not only be ineffectual but are even dangerous. According to considerable data, people popping vitamins C and E are predisposing themselves to cancer, according to a study published earlier this year in the journal *Stem Cells*, as high doses of these antioxidants can cause genetic abnormalities. Similarly, a study published in 2010 in the journal *Cancer Research* linked fish oil supplements with cancer in mice. Yet, the supplement craze goes on.

I can not afford to be a medical "best guesser" because my reputation and future patient care depends upon the accuracy of my data. Some things aren't researched because it isn't possible to do "gold standard" experiments, or because it isn't ethical to do them (i.e.: withholding lifesaving treatments to test if that will kill people). This is not the case with antioxidants and the data, utilizing randomized controlled trials (RCTs) as the gold standard, has shown their ineffectiveness and dangers.

Until other physicians read my books, they are merely guessing. It's educated guessing, but still guessing. They need to get the facts.

A good scientist knows the limits of his own knowledge. We don't have many open-minded scientists today. You don't get on TV or get the big grant money by saying, "I don't know," so they put on their best expert face and make things up. Does Dr. OoZe come to mind?

We need to rely on scientifically based evidence.

Although observational data from the general population has shown dietary antioxidant intake is associated with reduced disease incidence and morbidity and mortality, most clinical intervention trials have clearly failed to support this relationship.

The 15 dangers of using questionable antioxidant treatments include:
- overly optimistic expectations,

- an unsupported feeling of being treated effectively,
- delay in getting appropriate treatment,
- overall increase in mortality,
- increased risk of cancer,
- increased risk of heart disease,
- increased risk of stroke,
- decreased quality of life,
- direct physical harm,
- interference with proven treatment,
- being further misled with misinformation,
- waste of valuable time,
- financial harm,
- shortened life span
- and a host of other forms of damaging adverse effects.

Top Ten Things letting you know that you have been "radically misled" (duped) on the ruse of "beneficial" antioxidants:

1 - **The pinch your nose test** (you will die summarily without a constant supply of ground state triplet diradical oxygen)

2 - **The harmful effects of excessive endogenous antioxidants** (uric acid, cholesterol, bilirubin, estrogen, testosterone, steroids, etc.)

3 - **The 3 largest antioxidant studies were shut down early because it was unethical to continue knowingly harming the participants** (ATBC, CARET, SELECT)

4 - **The obvious benefits of excess EMODs** (exercise, hyperbaric oxygen, etc.)

5 - **Chronic granulomatous disease (CGD) patients clearly show the dangers of insufficient EMOD levels** (tumors, repeated infections, early deaths)

6 - **32 of the largest medical/scientific organizations do not recommend antioxidant use**

7 - **27 human cancer cell types shielded (protected) by antioxidants** (and 9 murine cancer cell types)

8 - **Harmful antioxidant study reports by categories** (hundreds of studies)

9 - A, C, E combinations and synergism increases their harmful effects (as opposed to making the antioxidants more effective)

10 - We humans do not synthesize the low molecular weight antioxidants (A, C & E), which are claimed to be of utmost importance. Why? (Aren't we at the top of the phylogenetic tree? or is Mother Nature just stupid?) This defies Darwinian principles. After millions of evolutionary years, mankind should have gotten it right by now.

Antioxidants lack supportive data

The mechanism of action of dietary antioxidants has not been established and most of the clinical studies are small. The effect of these antioxidants in protecting sperm from endogenous EMODs, gentle sperm processing and cryopreservation has not been established. (Zini et al, 2009)

Spermatozoa have little cytoplasmic fluid (antioxidant enzymes are generally intracellular), virtually no capacity for protein synthesis and little antioxidant capacity. (Zini et al, 1993)

There was no significant relationship between hormone concentrations, sperm DNA damage and total antioxidant capacity, suggesting other mechanisms for sperm dysfunction. (Appasamy et al, 2007)

No correlations were also found between DNA damage score and TAS, TOS levels and OSI in idiopathic infertile group. We did not find any relationship between sperm DNA damage and oxidative stress in normozoospermic infertile men. Verit et al think that the pathophysiology of idiopathic infertility cannot be explained by sperm DNA damage or seminal oxidative stress. (Verit et at, 2006)

To date, there are no studies to indicate a relationship between systemic antioxidant or vitamin deficiency and male infertility. Silver et al, 2005 evaluated a cohort of fertile men and did not identify any relationships between dietary antioxidant intake (vitamins C, E or ß-carotene) and sperm DNA damage. (Silver et al, 2005)

There was no dose-response association between any DNA fragmentation index (DFI) outcome and any antioxidant intake measure. (Silver et al, 2005)

No consistent associations were found between antioxidant or zinc intakes and sperm aneuploidy. (Young et al, 2008)

No significant changes in oocyte fertilization rate or embryo quality were detected between the Menevit antioxidant and the placebo groups. Side-effects on the Menevit antioxidant were rare (8%) and mild in nature. (Tremellen et al, 2007)

Antioxidants appear to be of limited value in protecting the DNA of normal spermatozoa from endogenous EMOD production (e.g. NADPH-induced or centrifugation-induced). (Twigg et al, 1998)

In general, antioxidants appear to be of limited value in protecting sperm DNA from gentle semen processing (e.g. incubation or density-gradient centrifugation). (Chi et al, 2008)

In some cases, antioxidant supplementation in vitro (e.g. combination of vitamins C and E) may cause sperm DNA damage. (Donnelly et al, 1999)

Addition of both ascorbate and alpha-tocopherol in combination to sperm preparation medium actually induced DNA damage and intensified the damage induced by H(2)O(2), however, H_2O_2-induced ROS production was significantly reduced in a dose-dependent manner by supplementation with both vitamins. (Donnelly et al, 1999)

Addition of glutathione and hypotaurine, either singly or in combination, to sperm preparation medium had no significant effect on sperm progressive motility or baseline DNA integrity. (Donnelly et al, 2000)

The mechanism of action of dietary antioxidants has not been established and most of the clinical studies are small. (Zini et al, 2009)

Ob-gyn guidelines often based on opinion, weak data

A September 2011 article stated solid evidence is often missing from the practice guidelines used by obstetrician-gynecologists across the U.S., a new study shows. **Less than a third of the recommendations from the American College of Obstetricians and Gynecologists (ACOG) are based on gold-standard scientific experiments**, researchers found. The rest are based on anecdotal evidence or expert opinion, which is subject to personal biases, they reported.

"That is often the fall-back when there is no data," said Dr. Andrew D. Auerbach, a professor of medicine at the University of California, San Francisco, who was not part of the study. He said expert opinion is helpful in pointing out what we don't know, but might not always translate into what's best for patients.

"Many, many times we have the best intentions and the best wishes and yet things don't work out the way we would have liked," Auerbach told Reuters Health. **Guidelines** help doctors keep up with the latest developments in their fields and are widely perceived as a recipe for good patient care.

But **there is often surprisingly little hard data behind them.** Earlier this year, for instance, **a group of researchers found that only one in seven treatment recommendations from the Infectious Diseases Society of America was based on high-quality data from clinical trials.**

One such recommendation urged doctors to treat pneumonia with antibiotics right away. It ended up fueling over treatment with no apparent benefits, possibly breeding resistant bacteria and exposing patients to side effects. (See Reuters Health story of January 10, 2011).

In the new study, Dr. Jason D. Wright of Columbia University in New York and colleagues went through **717 practice recommendations from ACOG, the nation's leading group of ob-gyns. They found 30 percent of those were based on top-notch evidence, so-called randomized controlled trials. About 38 percent came from observational studies, whose value is limited, and 32 percent were purely expert opinion.**

"It is disappointing, but I don't think it reflects their process," said Auerbach, who was recently part of an Institute of Medicine committee to develop standards for better guidelines. "It is really a call for better evidence."

In an editorial published along with the new study in ACOG's journal Obstetrics and Gynecology, Editor-in-Chief Dr. James R. Scott said **the group's guidelines compared favorably with those in other areas of medicine.**

He added that the guidelines panels conduct extensive reviews of the medical literature to find all relevant evidence and also take care to exclude experts with financial conflicts of interest.

According to Dr. Sheldon Greenfield, who chaired the Institute of Medicine guideline committee, those are two key elements in creating good guidelines. A third component is to ensure that guideline panels represent all stakeholders – including doctors from other specialties and patients, he told Reuters Health. If those requirements are fulfilled, he added, there is room for opinion.

"For many of the recommendations there simply is not enough data, or it is disputed," said Greenfield, a professor of medicine at the University of California, Irvine. "So there has to be a role for expert opinion."

So far, however, few if any guideline panels meet all three requirements. "It's about as common as peace in the Middle East," Greenfield said. "People are struggling with it."

SOURCE: http://bit.ly/pkPZu4 Obstetrics and Gynecology, September 2011.

Is Chemical in Plastic (BPA) Robbing Men of Sex Appeal?

According to Mikaela Conley, in a June 2011 article, a chemical found in common plastics may undermine a man's masculinity and his ability to attract a female, or at least that's what a new study on mice may suggest.

It is the latest research to question the health safety of the hormone-changing compound bisphenol-A, or BPA.

In the study, **researchers found that female mice were not attracted to male mice that were exposed to BPA in the womb.** They also noted that males exposed to the chemical in the womb were more likely to behave like females.

Researchers said female mice exposed to BPA were unaffected by the chemical.

It's possible that BPA exposure alters the males' hormone signals, researchers said, and some say the chemical exposure may have the same effect on people by altering developmental sexual traits in boys and girls.

"BPA has been shown to suppress the early production of testosterone. In short, the females can sense [the males'] compromised state and are less attracted to these males," said Cheryl Rosenfeld, associate professor in biomedical sciences at the University of Missouri and co-author of the study.

According to the Environmental Protection Agency, more than 1 million pounds of BPA are released into the environment each year, primarily used as an ingredient to harden plastic. The chemical has been widely scrutinized, causing several consumer products, including baby bottles, water bottles and microwavable dishware made with the compound, to be taken off the shelves.

Last year, the European Union and Canada banned the use of BPA in baby bottles. Many U.S. states are following suit by considering a ban on the chemical, as well.

Chemical in plastics (BPA) threatening masculinity?

The American Medical Association voted to adopt a policy which recognized BPA as a chemical that interferes with human hormones. The organization now urges makers of BPA plastics to label and identify the chemical in the product.

"While the exact outcomes may differ in humans, there is reason for concern that sex-specific behavioral alterations are a significant risk following prenatal exposure to BPA," said Dr. Rodney Dietert, professor of immunotoxicology at Cornell University. "Brain, behavior and immune effects are commonly seen with developmental exposure to BPA."

In a previous study, researchers linked BPA to lower sperm counts and smaller testes in male mice. Another study reported that a female mouse had reduced pregnancy rates when she mated with a male exposed to BPA, said Dr. John Spangler, associate professor at Wake Forest University School of Medicine.

"This study adds to the increasing evidence that BPA is a toxin that we should regulate more stringently," said Spangler.

Researchers said the mice were fed food laced with BPA at levels considered safe for human exposure, but the American Chemistry Council disagreed, saying "typical human exposures are miniscule compared to the dose used in the study."

"Given the incredibly high exposure levels of BPA used in this study—a single dose level approximately 250,000 times higher than typical human intake – there is little to be learned from the authors' work," the American Chemistry Council said in a statement.

The wide ranging harmful effects of antioxidants puts them in the "toxic" category and toxins do not belong in our food supply or ingestible from our environment.

"The government needs to take action."

"There is enough science here to show that these are potentially hazardous compounds and antioxidants shouldn't be in products that could lead to exposure to children."

I (RMH) have long been pushing for the federal government to regulate antioxidants, especially in children's products.

The FDA is sending dangerous mixed messages to the public about antioxidants.

CHAPTER NINE

The epiphany of 4-4-II

I believe that the antioxidant overkill is doing the following: the over supply of electrons by the electron donating antioxidants are allowing the 4 electron reduction of ground state oxygen (O_2) to proceed to the final step, i.e., the formation of water. In doing so, this, in effect, "removes" the spectacularly acting (more reactive) EMOD intermediates of superoxide, hydrogen peroxide, the hydroxyl radical, nitric oxide and peroxynitrite and "supplies" the non-reacting (non-protective) water to or within the milieu (intra- or extracellular). This, in effect, "quenches" the EMODs (ROS) and it also prevents the protective action (messaging) of the reactive EMODs against pathogens and cancer. This is an entirely new paradigm. This is how it is happening and explains the electron donating nature of the antioxidants and the electron accepting nature of oxygen. This explains "how" antioxidant overkill causes a harmful effect!!!!!

The antioxidant overload negates the beneficent actions of the intermediate EMODs. However, when the electron donating antioxidants are present in limited amounts, they serve as pre-oxidants or co-oxidants and form the active intermediates and reactive EMODs, after interacting with triplet oxygen. RMH

Finally, this explains the need for average amounts of antioxidants contained within a balanced nutritious diet, containing fresh fruits and vegetables. It also explains the failures of the antioxidant supplement studies, which were supplying an antioxidant overkill, thereby negating the protective EMOD effects against cancer and pathogens.

It has always puzzled me that antioxidants are "necessary" to form EMODs. In fact, this is why I referred to them as pre-oxidants or co-oxidants. The query for me was, "Then, how could the antioxidants be harmful?" Without them, ground state oxygen does not have an adequate source of available electrons to form the crucial reactive intermediate EMODs, i.e., the Ie (e, electron), 2e and 3e reduction products. But, with a sufficient amount of antioxidant electrons, oxygen can accept the electrons to form superoxide, hydrogen peroxide, the hydroxyl radical, nitric oxide and peroxynitrite (the active EMOD forms).

The basic redox chemistry is correct in that oxygen is the ultimate electron acceptor and antioxidants are the agents donating the electrons. This also explains the reason that transition metals, such as iron or copper, can also donate electrons to ground state oxygen and act as prooxidants. It is the antioxidant's contributions as electron donors that allows them to act to form the protective prooxidant EMOD intermediates.

Part of the problem is that our diet and our environment supply us with adequate (and sometimes over supply us) antioxidants. When we endeavor to "supplement" these sources, we overload the electron supply to oxygen and thus, it undergoes a 4 electron reduction to form water. Wow!!!! This is way cool. RMH 4-4-11

If you ride in a car,
you have an increased risk of being
in an automobile accident.
Now that's modern science at its finest, folks.
R. M. Howes, M.D., Ph.D.
2/26/11

THE SCIENTIFIC VOYAGER

The vast immensity of the data ocean surrounds
and engulfs you.
At first, you glimpse something foggy on the far
away research horizon.
You diligently pursue, in that direction, to get a better look.
A distant shape is then suggested, but needs
considerable clarification.

You move in, study it intensely - all possibilities, intensively.
An image of enlightenment begins to form.
It has a pattern and design....but is it real
or just another illusion?
More study, more study, more study and
now it congeals into focus. Your mind's eye
can see it ever so clearly.
It is a magnificent island of discovery
jutting out of a raging sea of unknowns.
Now, you must step out onto its slippery rock surface
to be scientifically satiated.
There....you feel it solidly under your feet. Eureka!
But how do you inform others of your discovery?
How do you bring them onshore with you?
Carefully, very, very carefully
for many are still blind,
still uninformed, still misinformed, still lost at sea!
Yet, for you, the tumultuous journey is at an end.
You are scientifically satisfied....
'till you launch the next inquiry.
R. M. Howes, M.D., Ph.D.
4/1/11

Male donors and female acceptors - a metaphor

Perhaps this is an appropriate place to introduce an appropriate sexual metaphor to describe oxidants and antioxidants.

Oxidants, such as oxygen, are electron acceptors and antioxidants are electron donors. Similarly, females are sperm acceptors and males are sperm donors.

There are spectra of acceptors from strong to weak and spectrums of donors from strong to weak. For instance, a manly man would be considered a strong donor and a wimpy man would be considered to be a weak donor.

Keeping the analogy going, once a female acceptor accepts the sperm, she becomes a weak donor (or male) and once the male donor donates his sperm, he becomes a weak acceptor (or female).

This transition explains why there is no "classic war game" between good (antioxidant donors) and bad (prooxidant acceptors). Once the electron exchange has occurred, they assume the role of their opposite counterpart. This is a very important concept to understand and it refutes the notion that antioxidants simply "mop up" or neutralize all of the bad prooxidants and ends the exchange of electrons or redox reactions.

The exchange of electrons is perpetuated until all reactants reach a condition of stable electron pairs and that does not happen in living biological systems. There is always a condition whereby electrons need to be transferred, e.g., a condition where electron flow (along with proton flow) is needed. Please remember, without electron and proton flow, we die summarily.

Additionally, certain molecules, especially transition metals, are designed to exist in varying electronic configuration states, which promotes electron and proton flow. That is what drives the whole biological system and the electron transport chain, the generation of energy and the flow of life.

That is precisely the way that we oxidatively produce energy and protect ourselves from pathogens and cancer.

It may be more apt to utilize a metaphor of a **hermaphrodite,** in which there can be leanings either towards the male or the female phenotype.

Vitamins C, E, A, and other antioxidants- male infertility

Vitamins C and E, as well as other agents such **as pentoxifylline and allopurinol are known to have antioxidant activity.** Reactive oxygen species are found at high levels in up to 40% of infertile men, whereas they are virtually never found in the semen of fertile men. **RMH Note:** But, is this a reaction to infertility or is it a cause of infertility?

Seminal fluid is known to be very rich in antioxidants, and removal of seminal fluid has an adverse action on sperm viability. In addition, vitamin C can decrease endogenous oxidative damage to sperm DNA after systemic administration to men. This activity was optimally seen at 250 mg/day of Vitamin C (the highest dose tested) and 400 IU (International Units) of Vitamin E, and especially in men who are predisposed to having low seminal fluid ascorbic acid levels, such as smokers.

However, **low levels of superoxide anion may be critically important to fertilization related events in sperm, including the acrosome reaction.**

And, it is possible that excessive levels of antioxidants may interfere with the acrosome reaction.

The adverse activity of some antioxidants, including pentox, on egg function may further support the physiologic action of low levels of some reactive oxygen species during fertilization.

In addition, no controlled studies have demonstrated a benefit of systemic administration of antioxidants on male fertility. Indeed, *one antioxidant, allopurinol, has been shown to have a specific drug-related effect on sperm function in a hamster-egg penetration test.*

High dose administration of antioxidants has theoretical adverse as well as potential beneficial effects on male fertility. **Use of these agents at pharmacologic doses should not be advocated until data exist to support their benefits in male infertility.**

No individual agent or agents can predictably improve sperm function or fertility for men with idiopathic subfertility. Prior to considering such nonspecific treatment, side effects, potential detrimental effects, and the paucity of documented benefit should be carefully presented to patients.

Based on these data, many generally recommend against empiric therapy to the infertility patients. Instead, specific interventions such as assisted reproduction that have a quantifiable benefit are suggested to the couple with idiopathic male infertility.

Spermatogenesis is an extremely active replicative process capable of generating approximately 1,000 sperm a second. The high rates of cell division inherent in this process **imply correspondingly high rates of mitochondrial oxygen consumption by the germinal epithelium.** However, the poor vascularization of the testes means that oxygen tensions in this tissue are low and that competition for this vital element within the testes is extremely intense.

Addition of glutathione and hypotaurine, either singly or in combination, to sperm preparation medium had no significant effect on sperm progressive motility or baseline DNA integrity. Despite this, sperm were still afforded significant protection against H_2O_2 induced damage and ROS generation. (Donnelly et al, 2000)

The mechanism of action of dietary antioxidants has not been established and most of the clinical studies are small. (Zini et al, 2009)

CHAPTER TEN

I present a summary of the important roles of EMODs in sexuality and reproduction.

CRUCIAL ROLE OF EMODs IN SEXUALITY: 22 items

- Spermatogenesis is an extremely active replicative process capable of generating approximately 1,000 sperm a second. The high rates of cell division inherent in this process imply correspondingly high rates of mitochondrial oxygen consumption by the germinal epithelium. However, the poor vascularization of the testes means that oxygen tensions in this tissue are low and that competition for this vital element within the testes is extremely intense.

- Addition of glutathione and hypotaurine, either singly or in combination, to sperm preparation medium had no significant effect on sperm progressive motility or baseline DNA integrity. Despite this, sperm were still afforded significant protection against H_2O_2 induced damage and ROS generation. (Donnelly et al, 2000) (Donnelly ET, et al. Glutathione and hypotaurine in vitro: effects on human sperm motility, DNA integrity and production of reactive oxygen species. Mutagenesis. 2000 Jan;15(1):61-8)

- The production of EMODs by sperm is a normal physiological process. (Sharma, Agarwal, 1996)

- Semen EMODs are generated by spermatozoa. (Aitken, Fisher, 1994)

- The controlled release of low levels of EMODs is necessary for normal sperm function. (Aitken, Fisher, 1994)

- Spermatozoa have little cytoplasmic fluid (antioxidant enzymes are generally intracellular), virtually no capacity for protein synthesis and little antioxidant capacity. (Zini et al, 1993)

RMH Note: If EMODs are harmful to spermatozoa, Darwinian principles suggest that sperm should have evolved adequate antioxidant defenses, but that has not occurred.

- Leukocytes and immature spermatozoa are the two main sources of ROS. (Garrido et al, 2004)

- In the reproductive tract, free radicals also play a dual role and can modulate various reproductive functions. (du Plessis et al, 2008)

- Controlled generation of EMODs has shown to be essential for the development of capacitation and hyperactivation, the two processes of sperm that are necessary to ensure fertilization. (de Lamirande, Gagnon, 1993)

- The axosome and associated dense fibers of the mid-piece in sperm are covered by mitochondria that generate energy (and EMODs) from intracellular stores of ATP depletion. (Bucak et al, 2008)

- Free radicals are also known as a necessary evil for intracellular signaling involved in the normal process of cell proliferation, differentiation, and migration of sperm. (Agarwal et al, 2004) (Rhee, 2006) (Ford, 2001)

- Physiological levels of EMODs influence and mediate the gametes. (Gagnon et al, 1991) (Aitken, 1997)) (Attaran et al, 2000) and crucial reproductive processes, such as sperm-oocyte interactions (de Lamirande et al, 1997), implantation and early embryo development. (Sakkas et al, 1998)

- EMODs generated by spermatozoa play an important role in normal physiological processes such as, sperm capacitation, acrosome reaction, maintenance of fertilizing ability, and stabilization of the mitochondrial capsule in the mid-piece in bovine. (Agarwal et al, 2008) (Goncalves et al, 2010) (Desai et al, 2009)

- Under physiological conditions, sperm produces small amounts of EMODs (ROS), which are needed for fertilization, acrosome reaction and capacitation.

- The mechanism of action of dietary antioxidants has not been established and most of the clinical studies are small. The effect of these antioxidants in protecting sperm from endogenous EMODs, gentle sperm processing and cryopreservation has not been established. (Zini et al, 2009)

- NOX enzymes are even involved in the respiratory burst that occurs during fertilization.

- Low levels of superoxide anion may be critically important to fertilization related events in sperm, including the acrosome reaction. And, it is possible that excessive levels of antioxidants may interfere with the acrosome reaction.

- Many evidences demonstrate that low and controlled concentrations of these ROS play an important role in sperm physiological processes such as capacitation, acrosome reaction, and signaling processes to ensure fertilization. (Bansal, Bilaspuri, 2010)

- Oxygen is instead used by a specific NADPH oxidase on the egg's surface for the purposeful production of nanomolar concentrations of hydrogen peroxide (Wong et al, 2004). Surprisingly, this burst of hydrogen peroxide production does not damage the nascent organism, but instead is used as part of an enzymatic reaction that ultimately results in the development of a protective shell around the young fertilized egg.

- ROS can be purposefully made and harnessed to regulate a diverse array of physiological processes. In turn, accumulating evidence also suggests that dysregulation of oxidant signaling may cause or accelerate a host of pathological conditions, including the rate that we age. Thus, seemingly from life's inception to its end, redox signaling acts as an important regulator of physiological and pathophysiological outcomes.

RMH Note: I believe that the fact that the zygote produces a hydrogen peroxide spike at conception, speaks volumes about the importance of EMODs in reproduction.

- Furthermore, the fact that bacteria and plants also heavily rely on aspects of oxidant signaling suggests that many of these mechanisms are ancient and evolutionarily conserved. A further understanding of these pathways promises to reveal to us many more secrets regarding how life begins, why it ends, and all the myriad complexities that make up the middle.

(Finkel, 2011)

- Penile erection is dependent upon vascular smooth muscle relaxation in erectile tissue and penile arteries, the principal mediator of relaxation being nitric oxide (NO).

THE CASE AGAINST ANTIOXIDANTS: 20 items

Because redox homeostasis presumably has a narrow biological window, it is conceivable that too much or too little oxidants (and antioxidants) could produce similar pathological effects.

- The adverse activity of some antioxidants, including pentox, on egg function may further support the physiologic action of low levels of some reactive oxygen species during fertilization.

- In addition, no controlled studies have demonstrated a benefit of systemic administration of antioxidants on male fertility. Indeed, *one antioxidant, allopurinol, has been shown to have a specific drug-related effect on sperm function in a hamster-egg penetration test.*

- High dose administration of antioxidants has theoretical adverse as well as potential beneficial effects on male fertility. Use of these agents at pharmacologic doses should not be advocated until data exist to support their benefits in male infertility.

- A definitive conclusion regarding the benefit of these therapies is difficult to obtain, as most of the previous studies lacked control groups, considered different antioxidants in different combinations and doses, or did not evaluate pregnancy rates in previously infertile couples.

- The exact mechanism of action of dietary antioxidants and the optimal dietary supplement have not been established. Moreover, most of the clinical studies are small and few have evaluated pregnancy rates. The effect of these antioxidants in protecting sperm from endogenous ROS, gentle sperm processing and cryopreservation has not been established conclusively. (Zini, Al-Hathal, 2011)

- No individual agent or agents can predictably improve sperm function or fertility for men with idiopathic subfertility.

- There was no significant relationship between hormone concentrations, sperm DNA damage and total antioxidant capacity, suggesting other mechanisms for sperm dysfunction. (Appasamy et al, 2007)

- Verit et al think that the pathophysiology of idiopathic infertility cannot be explained by sperm DNA damage or seminal oxidative stress. (Verit et at, 2006)

- To date, there are no studies to indicate a relationship between systemic antioxidant or vitamin deficiency and male infertility. Silver et al, 2005 evaluated a cohort of fertile men and did not identify any relationships between dietary antioxidant intake (vitamins C, E or ß-carotene) and sperm DNA damage. (Silver et al, 2005). I believe that this sums it up, in that there is no relationship between antioxidant supplement intake and prevention of DNA damage.

- There was no dose-response association between any DNA fragmentation index (DFI) outcome and any antioxidant intake measure. (Silver et al, 2005)

- No consistent associations were found between antioxidant or zinc intakes and sperm aneuploidy. (Young et al, 2008)

- No significant changes in oocyte fertilization rate or embryo quality were detected between the Menevit antioxidant and the placebo groups. Side-effects on the Menevit antioxidant were rare (8%) and mild in nature. (Tremellen et al, 2007)

- Antioxidants appear to be of limited value in protecting the DNA of normal spermatozoa from endogenous EMOD production (e.g. NADPH-induced or centrifugation-induced). (Twigg et al, 1998) (Cemeli et al, 2004) (Dobrzynska et al, 2004) (Anderson et al, 2003)

- In general, antioxidants appear to be of limited value in protecting sperm DNA from gentle semen processing (e.g. incubation or density-gradient centrifugation). (Chi et al, 2008) (Donnelley et al, 1999) (Hughes et al, 1998) (Donnelly et al, 2000)

- In some cases, antioxidant supplementation in vitro (e.g. combination of vitamins C and E) may cause sperm DNA damage. (Donnelly et al, 1999) (Hughes et al, 1998)

- *Addition of both ascorbate and alpha-tocopherol in combination to sperm preparation medium actually induced DNA damage and intensified the damage induced by* H_2O_2, however, H_2O_2-induced ROS production was significantly reduced in a dose-dependent manner by supplementation with both vitamins. (Donnelly et al, 1999)

- Addition of glutathione and hypotaurine, either singly or in combination, to sperm preparation medium had no significant effect on sperm progressive motility or baseline DNA integrity. Despite this, sperm were still afforded significant protection against H_2O_2 induced damage and ROS generation. (Donnelly et al, 2000)

- Before the end of the first trimester, 30%-50% of conceptions end in spontaneous abortion. Most losses occur at the time of implantation. 15%-20% of clinical pregnancies end in spontaneous abortions. Recurrent pregnancy loss is a frustrating clinical problem both for clinicians and patients. Recurrent pregnancy loss affects 0.5%-3% of women in the reproductive age group, and between 50%-60% of recurrent pregnancy losses are idiopathic.

- The role of antioxidant vitamins for primary prevention of oxidative stress-induced pathologies needs to be investigated further. (Gupta et al, 2007)

- Evidences have been reported that especially superoxide anion ($^{\bullet}O_2$) is required for the late stage of embryo development such as, two germ cell layers and egg cylinder. (Kodama et al, 1996)

CHAPTER ELEVEN

EMOD function

EMODs regulate vital pathways i.e., energy metabolism, survival/stress responses, apoptosis, inflammatory response, oxygen sensing, redox homeostasis, fertilization, survival kinase activation, ion channel regulation, apoptosis signaling, preconditioning, necrosis, inflammatory system, regulation of vascular tone, the activity of HIF (hypoxia inducible factor), etc.

An unavoidable and essential steady stream of EMODs emerge from our cellular factories to heal wounds, produce energy, detoxify harmful substances, and protect against pathogens and cancer.

As I have previously pointed out, in our bodies WBCs encounter pathogens and they literally shoot out a spike of hydrogen peroxide.

Free Radicals are molecules with an unpaired electron and are important intermediates in natural processes involving cytotoxicity, control of vascular tone, and neurotransmission. They are also responsible for some vital actions like destroying the bacteria and other cells of foreign matter, kill cancer cells, turning on and off of genes and fight infection, to keep our brain alert and in focus.

I am amazed that with the discovery of one antioxidant enzyme, SOD, scientists leaped up and hypothesized that this proved that SOD was there to overcome the deleterious effects of EMODs. Well, I submit that the multitude of oxidative enzymes (Duox, Fox, NADPH oxidase, NO synthase, MOA, mixed function oxidase, Cyt P450s, etc.) are proof that they are there to prevent the effects of antioxidant overloading, because of the combined effects of the endogenous antioxidant enzymes (SOD, catalase, GPx, etc.), endogenous antioxidants (uric acid, bilirubin, cholesterol, estrogens, testo-sterone, etc.) and ingestion of exogenous small molecular weight antioxidants (vitamins A, C and E, glutathione, selenium, etc.).

EMODs are formed via important biological systems, including the electron transport chain, NADPH oxidase, xanthine oxidase, prostaglandin synthe-sis, reduced riboflavin, nitric oxide synthetase, reperfusion injury, the cyto-chrome P450s, activated neutrophils and phagocytic cells. Outside sources of EMODs include drugs, antibiotics that depend on quinoid groups or bound metals for their action such as nitrofurantoin, and anti-cancer drugs such as doxorubicin, cisplatin, bleomycin and methotrexate, and pesticides, transition metals, tobacco smoke, alcohol, environmental radiation and high tempera-ture, radiation treatment, inhalation of inorganic particles such as asbestos and silica, and ozone inhalation and even fever.

NOX enzymes are even involved in the respiratory burst that occurs during fertilization. The biggest controllable EMOD source of all, behind normal breathing, is EXERCISE, which medical science has repeatedly validated is good for us.

Antioxidants block the good effects of exercise. All three layers of the vascu-lar wall [intima (i.e., endothelial cells), media (i.e., smooth muscle cells), and adventitia (i.e., fibroblasts and macrophages)] express NOX family members and all produce EMODs.

A failing dilated heart requires more oxygen per gram tissue than a non-failing smaller heart. I believe that this also means that it will be more susceptible to the decreasing levels of O_2, which are available to it, which are seen with aging and consequently, decreasing levels of EMODs are going to be produced, which will "allow" the progressive development of coronary atherosclerosis.

Although their role in the pathogenesis of clinical heart failure remains unclear, EMODs have been implicated by most authors to have a significant effect on cardiac function, including:

-hypertrophy
-ion flux and calcium handling
-EC coupling
-extracellular matrix configuration

-vasomotor function

-metabolism

-gene expression

-and downstream signaling of several growth factors and cytokines.

EMODs regulate several general classes of genes including:

-adhesion molecules and chemotactic factors

-antioxidant enzymes

-and vasoactive substances.

Our system of oxidative cure protects us from pathogenic agents such as:

- Bacteria

- Viruses

- Fungi

- Parasites

- Neoplasia

- Man's interventions (e.g., healers, shaman, physicians, gurus, medicinals, drugs, potions, elixirs, salves, sprays, douches, antibiotics, antioxidants, etc.)

- And it detoxifies pollutants, toxins and xenobiotics

H_2O_2 WES' H^IO_2LY GR$^I\Delta_g$IL

Bill Pryor et al wrote that the electronic ground state of dioxygen is a triplet ($^3O_2$). Since it has two unpaired electrons, both with the same spin, it also is a diradical. **The triplet state of oxygen (its ground state), $^3O_2$, acts as a diradical, a one-electron oxidant (albeit a fairly poor one),** whereas singlet $^1O_2$ acts as a more potent, often two-electron, oxidant that adds to π bonds, undergoes 'ene' reactions, and can insert into CH bonds.

The very existence of SOD implied a revolutionary concept. The notion that superoxide plays a role in biology and medicine **presupposes that oxygen, the prototypical oxidant in nature, can form superoxide, a species that usually reacts as a reductant.** In the mid-20th century when SOD was discovered, radicals were regarded as too reactive and unselective to play any role in biology.

(Radicals were thought to have a role that was limited to the chemistry that occurs in the stratosphere and in smog in the biosphere.) Radicals were believed to be too uncontrollable to occur in any reactions involving an enzyme; **radicals in cells were viewed as a "bull in a china shop."**

The 19th century literature on the "impossibility" of radicals existing in nature is amazing to read in the light of current knowledge illustrating the crucial role of EMODs in our very existence. **The mistaken belief that all radicals are extremely reactive and very short lived, led to the acceptance of the incorrect idea that radicals could not exist in vivo.** Another problem with the early analysis is the assumption that all radicals are "a bull in a china shop." In fact, radicals vary in reactivity (and therefore lifetimes) by some 10 orders of magnitude! Some radicals, such as the hydroxyl radical, react near the diffusion limit with the first molecule they bump into, whereas others, such as **semiquinones, are stable for days, weeks, or months.** So the "bull" may be reactive but also has his contemplative moments. **It was demonstrated that at least 40 various genes can be activated by H_2O_2 in mammalian cells.** The balance between oxidant production and antioxidant protection is believed to be critical in maintaining healthy biological systems. Therefore, **antioxidants at high doses could, despite acting as prooxidants, also disrupt the redox balance following their potential to interact with ROS (EMODs) present at physiological concentrations required for optimal cellular functioning, leading to cellular dysfunction.** This assumption was reinforced by findings showing that **transgenic animals overexpressing antioxidant enzyme systems (e.g., SOD and GPx) display abnormalities in function, including overexpression of certain genes such as immediate early genes (IEGs) and certain proteins. GPx overexpression in transgenic mice for example resulted in their development into a thermosensitive phenotype, suggesting a dysfunction in thermoregulation.**

Alleged EMOD damage - summary

Allegedly, EMODs (oxidative stress) have been hypothesized to cause the following damage:

- damage of the sperm plasma membrane
- cause a loss of DNA integrity
- lead to a failure of conception
- cause miscarriages

- cause spontaneous abortions
- cause idiopathic recurrent pregnancy loss
- cause hydatidiform mole
- cause defective embryogenesis
- cause drug-induced teratogenicity
- cause oxidant-induced endothelial damage, impaired placental vascularization and immune malfunction
- cause multifactorial and polygenic etiologies of abortion, recurrent pregnancy loss and defective embryogenesis
- cause intrauterine growth restriction and fetal dysmorphogenesis
- oxidant stress has been linked to the formation of antiphospholipid antibodies in the antiphospholipid syndrome
- may even cause childhood cancer
- cause male infertility
- cause sperm dysfunction
- reduce male reproductive potential
- cause endometriosis, ovarian cancer, and polycystic ovary disease via proinflammatory cytokines
- male and female infertility, including fetal dysmorphogenesis, abortions, and intrauterine growth restriction
- damage spermatogenesis and Leydig cell steroidogenesis
- cause erectile dysfunction (ED)
- and finally, (and allegedly), peroxidative damage is currently regarded as the single most important cause of impaired testicular function underpinning the pathological consequences of a wide range of conditions from testicular torsion to diabetes and xenobiotic exposure.

Before the end of the first trimester, 30%-50% of conceptions end in spontaneous abortion. Most losses occur at the time of implantation. 15%-20% of clinical pregnancies end in spontaneous abortions. Recurrent pregnancy loss is a frustrating clinical problem both for clinicians and patients. Recurrent pregnancy loss affects 0.5%-3% of women in the reproductive age group, and between 50%-60% of recurrent pregnancy losses are idiopathic.

The role of antioxidant vitamins for primary prevention of oxidative stress-induced pathologies needs to be investigated further. (Gupta et al, 2007)

One must use extreme care when altering antioxidant defenses. The redox balance is a critical aspect of all aerobic life. EMODs are signaling mechanisms for a vast range of vital metabolic pathways and networks, including those involved in sexual performance. Penile erection is dependent upon vascular smooth muscle relaxation in erectile tissue and penile arteries, the principal mediator of relaxation being the radical, nitric oxide (NO). RMH Note: This free radical response can be theoretically blocked by antioxidants.

However, increased inactivation of NO by superoxide results in impaired penile NO transmission and smooth muscle relaxation. Furthermore, propagation of endothelial dysfunction by ROS may result in chronic impairment of penile vascular function, a process analogous to early atherogenesis. Indeed, ED and atherosclerosis are closely linked through shared risk factors. (Jones et al, 2002)

Under physiological conditions, sperm produces small amounts of EMODs (ROS), which are needed for fertilization, acrosome reaction and capacitation. However, if an increased production of EMODs is not associated with a similar increase in scavenging systems, peroxidative damage of the sperm plasma membrane and loss of DNA integrity typically occur, which leads to cell death and reduced fertility. Furthermore, since there is no linear correlation between sperm quality and pregnancy rates, an improvement in semen parameters should not be the sole outcome considered in studies of antioxidant therapies. A definitive conclusion regarding the benefit of these therapies is difficult to obtain, as most of the previous studies lacked control groups, considered different antioxidants in different combinations and doses, or did not evaluate pregnancy rates in previously infertile couples. Even if beneficial effects were reported in a few cases of male infertility, more multi-center, double-blind studies performed with the same criteria are necessary for an increased understanding of the effects of various antioxidants on fertility. (Lombardo et al, 2011)

The exact mechanism of action of dietary antioxidants and the optimal dietary supplement have not been established. Moreover, most of the clinical studies are small and few have evaluated pregnancy rates. The effect of these antioxidants in protecting sperm from endogenous ROS, gentle sperm processing and cryopreservation has not been established conclusively. (Zini, Al-Hathal, 2011)

Pomegranate extract significantly improved intracavernosal blood flow, erectile activity, smooth muscle relaxation and fibrosis of the atherosclerotic group in comparison with the atherosclerotic group receiving placebo, but **did not normalize them to the age-matched control levels.** (Zhang et al, 2011)

Hypercholesterolemia is an example of antioxidant overkill and it causes erectile dysfunction.

CHAPTER TWELVE

I need to present a summary of the role of EMODs and antioxidants in sexual function. EMODs are essential at various stages of reproduction as follows:

EMODs, oxygen free radicals (ROS) and normal sperm

The production of EMODs is a normal physiological process.

Many evidences demonstrate that low and controlled concentrations of these ROS play an important role in sperm physiological processes such as capacitation, acrosome reaction, and signaling processes to ensure fertilization. (Bansal, Bilaspuri, 2010)

The production of EMODs by sperm is a normal physiological process. (Sharma, Agarwal, 1996)

EMODs generated by spermatozoa play an important role in normal physiological processes such as, sperm capacitation, acrosome reaction, maintenance of fertilizing ability, and stabilization of the mitochondrial capsule in the mid-piece in bovine. (Agarwal et al, 2008) (Goncalves et al, 2010) (Desai et al, 2009)

Evidences have been reported that especially superoxide anion $(^{\bullet}O_2)$ is required for the late stage of embryo development such as, two germ cell layers and egg cylinder. (Kodama et al, 1996)

Controlled generation of EMODs has shown to be essential for the development of capacitation and hyperactivation, the two processes of sperm that are necessary to ensure fertilization. (de Lamirande, Gagnon, 1993)

The axosome and associated dense fibers of the mid-piece in sperm are covered by mitochondria that generate energy (and EMODs) from intracellular stores of ATP depletion. (Bucak et al, 2008)

Free radicals are also known as a necessary evil for intracellular signaling involved in the normal process of cell proliferation, differentiation, and migration of sperm. (Agarwal et al, 2004) (Rhee, 2006) (Ford, 2001)

Physiological levels of EMODs influence and mediate the gametes. (Gagnon et al, 1991) (Aitken, 1997) (Attaran et al, 2000) and crucial reproductive processes, such as sperm-oocyte interactions (de Lamirande et al, 1997), implantation and early embryo development. (Sakkas et al, 1998)

Semen EMODs are generated by spermatozoa. (Aitken, Fisher, 1994)

The controlled release of low levels of EMODs is necessary for normal sperm function. (Aitken, Fisher, 1994)

In the reproductive tract, free radicals also play a dual role and can modulate various reproductive functions. (du Plessis et al, 2008)

Leukocytes and immature spermatozoa are the two main sources of ROS. (Garrido et al, 2004)

Levels of EMODs may rarely fluctuate within a fertile individual, but, do not affect sperm concentration and motility. (Bansal, Bilaspuri, 2010)

The physiological balance of reactive oxygen species (ROS) is ultimately determined by the rate of O_2^- production, the metabolism rate of O_2^- by endogenous superoxide dismutases (SODs), and the removal rate of H_2O_2 via antioxidant enzymes (catalase or glutathione peroxidase) and/or involvement in Haber-Weiss or Fenton chemistry. (Adler et al., 1999) (Haddad et al., 2002) (Miller et al., 2006)

In mammalian cells, potential enzymatic O_2^- sources include the mitochondrial electron-transport chain, the arachidonic acid-metabolizing enzymes (cyclooxygenase and lipoxygenase), the cytochrome P450s, xanthine oxidase, NADPH-oxidases, and NO synthases. (Babior et al., 1999) (Griendling et al., 1999) (Van Heerebeek et al., 2002) (Ogawa et al., 2003) (Genova et al., 2004)

Among these, the NADPH-oxidases (NOX) and cyclooxygenases / lipoxygenases are generally recognized as the principal physiological sources of O_2^-, which is in turn dismutated into H_2O_2. (Babior et al., 1999) (Griendling et al., 1999) (Van Heerebeek et al., 2002) (Kuhn et al., 1999) (Rhee et al., 2003)

H_2O_2 is now generally believed to be one of the most important ROS molecules in the modulation of multiple cellular events, including receptor-mediated signaling, apoptosis, proinflammation, and metabolism. (Davies et al., 1999) (Lee et al., 1999) (Aslan et al., 2003) (Tonks et al., 2005) (Saito et al, 2006)

EMODs (electronically modified oxygen derivatives, formerly called reactive oxygen species, ROS)

Antioxidants: Are they protectors?

The association between sperm DNA damage and semen EMODs is the basis for the use of antioxidants in the treatment of sperm DNA damage. High levels of EMODs have been detected in the semen of 25% of infertile men. (Iwasaki, Gagnon, 1992) (Zini et al, 1993)

The mechanism of action of dietary antioxidants has not been established and most of the clinical studies are small. A beneficial effect of in vitro antioxidant supplements in protecting sperm DNA from exogenous oxidants has been demonstrated, however, the effect of these antioxidants in protecting sperm from endogenous EMODs, gentle sperm processing and cryopreservation has not been established. (Zini et al, 2009)

Seminal fluid is an important source of antioxidants (ROS, EMOD scavengers) and is key in protecting spermatozoa from oxidative injury. (Jeulin et al, 1989) (Gagnon et al, 1991) (Zini et al, 1993)

Spermatozoa have little cytoplasmic fluid (antioxidant enzymes are generally intracellular), virtually no capacity for protein synthesis and little antioxidant capacity. (Zini et al, 1993)

RMH Note: If EMODs are harmful to spermatozoa, Darwinian principles suggest that sperm should have evolved adequate antioxidant defenses, but that has not occurred.

The endogenous free radical scavenging enzymes in the male reproductive tract include superoxide dismutase (SOD), catalase, and glutathione peroxidase (GPx). (Zini et al, 1993) (Zini et al, 1996) (Zini, Schlegel, 1997) (Jow et al, 1993) (Zini et al, 1997)

These same antioxidant enzymes (SOD, catalase and GPx) are found in semen. (Sanocka et al, 1997)

Several non-enzymatic antioxidants (e.g. vitamins C and E, hypotaurine, taurine, L-carnitine, lycopene) are also found in semen and this non-enzymatic component accounts for much of the total seminal antioxidant activity. (Holmes et al, 1992) (Zini et al, 1993)

There was no significant relationship between hormone concentrations, sperm DNA damage and total antioxidant capacity, suggesting other mechanisms for sperm dysfunction. (Appasamy et al, 2007)

No correlations were also found between DNA damage score and TAS, TOS levels and OSI in idiopathic infertile group. We did not find any relationship between sperm DNA damage and oxidative stress in normozoospermic infertile men. Verit et al think that the pathophysiology of idiopathic infertility cannot be explained by sperm DNA damage or seminal oxidative stress. (Verit et at, 2006)

To date, there are no studies to indicate a relationship between systemic antioxidant or vitamin deficiency and male infertility. Silver et al, 2005 evaluated a cohort of fertile men and did not identify any relationships between dietary antioxidant intake (vitamins C, E or ß-carotene) and sperm DNA damage. (Silver et al, 2005). I believe that this sums it up, in that there is no relationship between antioxidant supplement intake and prevention of DNA damage.

There was no dose-response association between any DNA fragmentation index (DFI) outcome and any antioxidant intake measure. (Silver et al, 2005)

No consistent associations were found between antioxidant or zinc intakes and sperm aneuploidy. (Young et al, 2008)

No significant changes in oocyte fertilization rate or embryo quality were detected between the Menevit antioxidant and the placebo groups. *Side-effects on the Menevit antioxidant were rare (8%) and mild in nature.* But, the Menevit antioxidant appears to be a useful ancillary treatment that significantly improves pregnancy rates in couples undergoing IVF-ICSI treatment for severe male factor infertility. (Tremellen et al, 2007)

Antioxidants appear to be of limited value in protecting the DNA of normal spermatozoa from endogenous EMOD production (e.g. NADPH-induced or centrifugation-induced). (Twigg et al, 1998) (Cemeli et al, 2004) (Dobrzynska et al, 2004) (Anderson et al, 2003)

In general, antioxidants appear to be of limited value in protecting sperm DNA from gentle semen processing (e.g. incubation or density-gradient centrifugation). (Chi et al, 2008) (Donnelley et al, 1999) (Hughes et al, 1998) (Donnelly et al, 2000)

In some cases, antioxidant supplementation in vitro (e.g. combination of vitamins C and E) may cause sperm DNA damage. (Donnelly et al, 1999) (Hughes et al, 1998)

Addition of both ascorbate and alpha-tocopherol in combination to sperm preparation medium actually induced DNA damage and intensified the damage induced by H_2O_2 *however,* H_2O_2-induced ROS production was significantly reduced in a dose-dependent manner by supplementation with both vitamins. (Donnelly et al, 1999)

Addition of glutathione and hypotaurine, either singly or in combination, to sperm preparation medium had no significant effect on sperm progressive motility or baseline DNA integrity. Despite this, sperm were still afforded significant protection against H_2O_2 induced damage and ROS generation. (Donnelly et al, 2000)

The mechanism of action of dietary antioxidants has not been established and most of the clinical studies are small. (Zini et al, 2009)

CHAPTER THIRTEEN

Signal transduction by reactive oxygen species

Although historically viewed as purely harmful, recent evidence suggests that **reactive oxygen species (ROS) function as important physiological regulators of intracellular signaling pathways. The specific effects of ROS are modulated in large part through the covalent modification of specific cysteine residues found within redox-sensitive target proteins.** Oxidation of these specific and reactive cysteine residues in turn can lead to the reversible modification of enzymatic activity. **Emerging evidence suggests that EMODs regulate diverse physiological parameters ranging from the response to growth factor stimulation to the generation of the inflammatory response**, and that dysregulated ROS signaling may contribute to a host of human diseases. (Finkel, 2011)

Introduction

Very early in his career, while working in a remote marine biological laboratory in 1908 in Italy, the young Otto Warburg observed that fertilization of sea urchin eggs resulted in a rapid and nearly sixfold increase in oxygen consumption. The notion that oxygen consumption was dynamic and seemingly tied to cellular proliferation would have a profound effect on the young scientist. Later, these ideas would be refined and focused not on normal fertilization but rather on the metabolic abnormalities of cancer cells.

Some 23 years after his observations in Italy, Warburg was awarded the Nobel Prize for his discovery of the "nature and mode of action of the respiratory enzyme." Interestingly, although Warburg's oocyte observations have been confirmed by many others, his hypothesis that this represented a burst of mitochondrial oxidative phosphorylation is undoubtedly incorrect. Indeed, nearly 100 years after his initial observation, it was established that the surge of oxygen consumption after fertilization is not, as originally envisioned, some primitive metabolic wakeup call by the young zygote. Rather, in 2004, Wong believed **oxygen is instead used by a specific NADPH oxidase on the egg's surface for the purposeful production of nanomolar concentrations of hydrogen peroxide.**

Surprisingly, this burst of hydrogen peroxide production does not damage the nascent organism, but instead is used as part of an enzymatic reaction that ultimately results in the development of a protective shell around the young fertilized egg.

These observations are in concert with a growing body of evidence that suggests that **ROS can be purposefully made and harnessed to regulate a diverse array of physiological processes.** In turn, accumulating evidence in 2005 by Balaban et al. also suggests that dysregulation of oxidant signaling may cause or accelerate a host of pathological conditions, **including the rate that we age.** Thus, **seemingly from life's inception to its end, redox signaling acts as an important regulator of physiological and pathophysiological outcomes.**

Oxidants and their cellular targets

There are numerous potential sources of ROS within the cell. As mentioned above, **one important generator of intracellular oxidants is a family of membrane-bound enzymes that rely on NADPH for their activity.** Although the expression of these enzymes was initially thought to be confined to phagocytic cells, it now appears that this seven-member family (Nox1–5 and Duox1–2) is in fact widely expressed and evolutionarily conserved.

To date, **the only clear function of these NADPH-dependent oxidases is the regulated generation of ROS. Mitochondria represent another source for intracellular oxidant production.** Most evidence suggests that mitochondrial oxidants are formed predominantly at complex I or complex III of the cytochrome chain when electrons initially derived from NADH or $FADH_2$ can react with oxygen to produce superoxide anions.

Although one-electron reactions predominate, two-electron reactions that allow the direct reduction of molecular oxygen to hydrogen peroxide do exist within the mitochondria. The fraction of total oxygen consumption that is diverted into mitochondrial ROS production is a difficult number to accurately estimate.

Although in isolated mitochondria under nonphysiological conditions this fraction can approach two percent or more, in the in vivo situation, the fraction of oxygen diverted to ROS production is presumably significantly less. In addition to the mitochondria and NADPH oxidases, **additional cellular sources of ROS production include a host of other intracellular enzymes such as xanthine oxidase, cyclooxygenases, cytochrome p450 enzymes, and lipoxygenases that produce oxidants as part of their normal enzymatic function.**

Reactive **oxygen species generation and disposal in the mitochondria.** Primary sources of ROS occur from the transfer of electrons (e^-) to molecular oxygen at either Complex I or III. Superoxide produced at Complex I is thought to form only within the matrix, whereas at Complex III superoxide is released both into the matrix and the inner mitochondrial space (IMS). In addition to the cytochrome chain, ROS can be formed by enzymatic action of numerous enzymes including monoamine oxidase (MAO) and cytochrome b_5 reductase (Cb_5R) located on the outer mitochondrial membrane (OMM), as well as glycerol-3-phosphate dehydrogenase (GPDH) and in some cell types, various cytochrome P450 enzymes located in the inner mitochondrial membrane (IMM). There are also several matrix enzymes and complexes (box) including aconitase, pyruvate dehydrogenase (PDH), and α-ketoglutarate dehydrogenase (αKGDH) that can generate superoxide. **Although one-electron reactions predominate, two-electron reactions leading to direct hydrogen peroxide production can occur as when, for instance, cytochrome c (Cyt C) and p66shc interact within the IMS.** Once generated, superoxide is dismutated spontaneously or enzymatically by manganese superoxide dismutase (MnSOD). **The hydrogen peroxide that is formed is further catabolized by the action of enzymes such as catalase (CAT), glutathione peroxidase (GPx), and peroxiredoxin 3 (Prx3).**

Although it had been appreciated for some time that mitochondria produced ROS as part of aerobic respiration and that phagocytic cells could produce oxidants as part of a host defense mechanism, the role of oxidants within cells began to shift with the observation that the production of hydrogen peroxide was essential for normal growth factor signaling.

These studies demonstrated that for growth factors such as PDGF and EGF, ligand binding stimulated a burst of ROS production. Inhibiting this rise in

ROS levels was shown to block the normal tyrosine kinase signaling induced by growth factor addition. These initial reports speculated that the intracellular target of oxidants might be the family of tyrosine and dual specific phosphatases, a hypothesis that was subsequently elegantly established.

The basis for this regulation of phosphatase activity centers on the unique chemistry of certain reactive cysteine residues. Although the pKa of thiol group on free cysteine is between 8 and 9, in some tyrosine phosphatases or similar target molecules, the surrounding amino acid microenvironment of the cysteine can be substantially modified to result in pKas as low as 4 to 5. These reactive cysteine residues are easily oxidized to a sulfenic form (RSOH). The sulfenic form is unstable and can undergo further oxidation via disproportionation to a sulfinic (RSO_2H) species.

Under greater oxidative stress, the sulphonic (RSO_3H) species can be created. Other possibilities for post-translational cysteine modifications include nitrosylation (RSNO), glutathionylation (RSSG), or the formation of an inter- or intramolecular disulfide bond (RSSR). Although reactive cysteine residues have long been identified experimentally using individual purified proteins, the ability to predict these residues based on either computational means or through large-scale proteomic approaches is a relatively recent development. **These more recent analysis has suggested that reactive and potentially modulatory cysteine residues might exist in well over 500 individual proteins, thereby extending this form of redox regulation to a wide range of enzymatic activities.**

Cysteine **biochemistry allows for redox-dependent signaling.** Specific reactive cysteine (Cys) residues within target proteins can be covalently modified by oxidative stress. Much like phosphorylation on serine or threonine residues, alteration of the thiol group can in turn modify enzymatic activity. Although the sulfenic form (SOH) is readily reversible, higher states of oxidation generally, but not always, lead to irreversible modification.

Although such analysis has established a role for intracellular oxidants in signal transduction, given the wide range of putative targets and the general reactivity of hydrogen peroxide, how can any specificity be achieved? At this point, this remains an open and potentially vexing concern.

Part of the answer may however result from the colocalization of the source of oxidant production nearby to the intended target. A 2010 report by Woo et al. demonstrated this principle by analyzing the antioxidant peroxiredoxin I (PrxI), which was transiently phosphorylated on a tyrosine residue after growth factor stimulation. This phosphorylation only occurred on a relatively small fraction of PrxI molecules, especially that fraction of PrxI located near the membrane oxidant source and nearby various membrane-associated signaling intermediates.

Phosphorylation of PrxI actually inhibited the antioxidant function of the protein, thereby allowing for the local accumulation of ROS near the membrane and presumably allowing for cysteine modification confined to this local area beneath the growth factor receptor. **Another 2009 study by Niethammer et al. using a zebrafish model visually identified a gradient of hydrogen peroxide levels within tissue that was essential for signaling.** It should be noted that in both preceding examples, the source of oxidants appeared to be a member of the Nox family of membrane-bound NADPH oxidases. These enzymes produce extracellular superoxide anions. It is generally believed that for signaling purposes, the superoxide anion dismutates spontaneously to hydrogen peroxide.

Although it had been generally assumed that once generated, hydrogen peroxide could simply diffuse back across the plasma membrane, recent evidence suggests that hydrogen peroxide might preferentially enter the cell through specific plasma membrane aquaporin channels. This regulated entry provides another potential mechanism through which oxidants could be channeled to an intended target and thereby achieve some measure of overall signaling specificity.

Extracellular oxidants are channeled back into the cell through specific plasma membrane aquaporins. Although hydrogen peroxide can be rapidly and efficiently degraded by intracellular antioxidants, Src family members stimulated by growth factors appear to phosphorylate and subsequently inactivate the main intracellular peroxide scavenger, peroxiredoxin (Prx I). **This PrxI inactivation only occurs in the region surrounding the stimulated growth factor, thus allowing for the local accumulation of hydrogen peroxide.** When the ROS reach sufficient levels, target molecules such as protein phosphatases (PTP) can be reversibly oxidized.

Antioxidants and signaling

The maintenance of intracellular redox homeostasis is dependent on a complex web of antioxidant molecules. These antioxidants include low molecular weight molecules such as **glutathione, present in millimolar concentrations within cells,** as well as an array of protein antioxidants that each have specific subcellular localizations and chemical reactivities. Included among the protein antioxidants are molecules such as superoxide dismutase that reacts with superoxide and **catalase and the peroxiredoxins that catabolize hydrogen peroxide.**

In addition, the thioredoxin and glutaredoxin family of proteins play a significant role in maintaining redox homeostasis by the reduction of disulfide bridges in various target proteins. It was proposed in 2011 by Jones and Go that these various protein antioxidants might exist in some loose hierarchical network or redox circuit, whose function is to maintain the overall cysteine proteome.

One of the earliest descriptions of this trend emerged from the **One important and emerging theme is that antioxidant proteins are not merely passive disposers of intracellular oxidants but rather active participants in redox signaling** interaction between thioredoxin (Trx) and the apoptosis signal–regulating kinase (ASK1). It had been previously known that agents such as TNF that activate ASK1 also stimulate ROS production.

Furthermore, it was known that ASK1 regulates the induction of downstream effectors such as the c-Jun N-terminal kinase (JNK) and the p38 MAPK pathway required for cell death. The link between ROS production and the subsequent activation of ASK1-dependent signaling appears to involve a redox-dependent interaction between ASK1 and Trx. In this model, oxidative stress leads to the direct oxidation of Trx and its subsequent dissociation from ASK1. Freed from the interaction with Trx, ASK1 can now activate its downstream target. **Importantly, in this scenario, Trx acts less as a classical antioxidant, and more as a sensor of intracellular oxidants and a regulator of redox signaling.**

I believe that this is supportive of my concept that antioxidants can serve as co-oxidants or pre-oxidants.

Antioxidant proteins can regulate signaling pathways. Proteins like thioredoxin (Trx) can function in cells to maintain redox balance by catalyzing the reduction of oxidized proteins (top). Trx can in turn be reduced through a process involving thioredoxin reductase and NADPH. In addition, Trx can also participate in redox signaling by directly binding to signaling intermediates such as ASK1 (bottom). In this case, the TrxI–ASK1 interaction is redox dependent and in turn modulates the capacity of ASK1 to activate downstream effectors such as p38 MAPK and the c-Jun N-terminal kinase (JNK).

The peroxiredoxins represent another family of antioxidant proteins that appear to directly modulate signaling within cells. Originally isolated in yeast, **the peroxiredoxins are abundant proteins that catalyze the reduction of hydrogen peroxide using an active site reactive cysteine.**

There are at least six different peroxiredoxin mammalian isoforms, each with slightly different subcellular localization and enzymatic mechanisms. Similar to what has been described with Trx and Nrx, members of the peroxiredoxin family appear to function not as simple antioxidants but rather they appear to bind and regulate a host of other molecules. For instance, peroxiredoxin I (PrxI) can bind to and modulate the activity of the androgen receptor, the cellular proto-oncogene c-Abl, and the stress kinase JNK.

Furthermore, 2009 evidence by Cao et al. suggests that PrxI can associate with the lipid phosphatase PTEN. Consistent with these latter observations, PrxI appears to act as a bone fide tumor suppressor as whole body or conditional PrdxI knockout mice exhibit altered PTEN activity with a resulting increased rate of tumor formation.

Perhaps the most startling nontraditional antioxidant function of the per-oxiredoxins came from recent observations linking this family to circadian rhythms. Previous work on biological clocks had established a pattern of gene and protein expression that occurs with a 24-h oscillating fashion. These studies have shown that such circadian rhythms are largely maintained by a nuclear transcriptional–translational feedback system whereby key clock proteins feedback to negatively regulate their own transcription. However, observations in some simple bacteria challenged the assumption that circadian cycles always required transcription and translation.

In a 2011 set of observations by O'Neill and Reddy, these notions were further advanced by studying red blood cells (RBCs) from human volunteers. The mature RBC is unique in the human body as it lacks a nucleus and therefore is incapable of new RNA production. **Surprisingly, when isolated from volunteers and maintained in culture, human RBCs exhibited a circadian oscillation of peroxiredoxin oxidation and reduction.** Remarkably, the sulfinic form of Prx undergoes rhythmic oscillation for several days in culture. These results again underscore the notion that **oxidants are intricately coupled to the regulation of crucial physiological processes and that antioxidants such as peroxiredoxin are not merely scavengers but rather exist in the cell as sensors and effectors of key redox-regulated pathways.**

Finally, it is important to note that **there is growing evidence that the regulation of antioxidant levels in cells is intimately tied to the levels of intracellular ROS and sources of oxidant production.** A well-studied example of this phenomenon is the Nrf2 transcription factor that regulates the expression of a host of antioxidant and detoxifying genes by binding to promoter sequences containing a consensus antioxidant response element.

In turn, the subcellular localization and hence activity of Nrf2 is at least in part regulated by its interaction with an inhibitory protein called KeapI. Specific reactive cysteine residues on KeapI are required for this regulation. A similar situation exists for the FoxO family of transcription factors that alter their subcellular localization based on the intracellular redox state and in turn, regulate the expression of various antioxidant genes.

This phenomenon also extends to ROS-producing organelles. In mammals, mitochondrial biogenesis, the physiological induction of new mitochondria, is regulated by the transcriptional coactivator PGC-Ialpha. Interestingly, PGC-Ialpha appears to regulate new mitochondrial formation while simultaneously regulating antioxidant expression.

This coordination of new ROS-producing organelles with increased antioxidant levels presumably helps maintain redox homeostasis. Although PGC-Ialpha is not present in lower organisms, it would appear that in yeast, the release of mitochondrial ROS can also act as signal to regulate the formation of new mitochondria. **Such results again suggest a coupling between mitochondrial number, oxidant production, and the antioxidant network.**

Oxidative stress and human disease

Although the preceding discussion revolved mostly around the role of ROS in normal physiological signaling, **growing evidence implicates alterations in redox signaling as a contributor to many disease processes.** Nonetheless, the precise role that oxidants play remains controversial and often beset with the problem as to whether a rise in ROS causes or merely correlates with the disease state.

Although an exhaustive description of the involvement of redox signaling in human disease is beyond the scope of this review, I will briefly highlight a few illustrative examples that exemplify some of the general principles.

The development of insulin resistance and subsequent type 2 diabetes mellitus (T2DM) is one area where oxidants have been consistently implicated in disease pathogenesis. Cellular models of insulin resistance are characterized by persistently elevated ROS levels.

Although these data suggest that high levels of ROS contribute to insulin resistance, there are other datasets that suggest the complete opposite might be true. For instance, **there is some evidence that mitochondrial oxidants are required for the glucose-induced insulin secretion by pancreatic beta-cells.** Furthermore, like many other growth factors, **insulin binding to its cell surface receptor stimulates production of hydrogen peroxide.** This rise in ROS levels has been shown to be necessary for the transient inactivation of protein tyrosine phosphatases such as PTP1B and TC45. As such, **ROS are also necessary to maintain normal insulin sensitivity.**

This point was underscored recently by the demonstration that mice lacking the antioxidant glutathione peroxidase showed higher ROS levels, leading to the inactivation of the lipid phosphatase PTEN. This phosphatase inactivation resulted in higher PI3-K/Akt signaling in these animals and improved insulin sensitivity. In these animals, treatment with an antioxidant actually made the glucose metabolism worse. Analysis of rare individuals with selenoprotein deficiency suggests that these observations may potentially extend to humans as well.

Presently, it is far from clear as to why in certain cellular and animal models, insulin resistance is associated with increased ROS levels and scavenging these oxidants improves metabolic homeostasis, whereas **in other models high ROS levels are associated with improved insulin sensitivity and antioxidants make things worse.** Possible explanations include differences in the intensity and sources of oxidants, a change in the function of oxidants depending on the stage of the disease, as well as specific but potentially important differences in the various metabolic models used.

In addition, **because redox homeostasis presumably has a narrow biological window, it is conceivable that too much or too little oxidants (and antioxidants) could produce similar pathological effects.**

Aging is another arena in which the role of oxidants has been often implicated but never definitively established. There is a long history, first formally articulated by Denham Harman in 1956, suggesting that the production of reactive oxygen species was linked to the rate of aging.

Indeed, there is a large body of mostly correlative literature suggesting that aging is accompanied by an increase in the steady-state level of oxidants and oxidatively modified proteins, lipids, and DNA. Consistent with a causal role for oxidants, in some lower organisms and mammalian models, increasing the level of antioxidants results in life span extension. In addition, certain long-lived mouse models such as deletion of the p66shc gene appear to extend life by modulating ROS levels.

In contrast, there are other models in lower organisms whereby the addition of low levels of ROS-producing compounds actually extends life, and where the genetic reduction of antioxidant defenses actually promotes a longer lifespan. These effects have also been observed at the cellular level and are generally ascribed to the concept of mitochondria, the biological equivalent of Fredrick Nietzsche dictum, "what won't kill you, will make you strong."

Finally, it should be noted that in some mouse models, reducing or increasing scavenging capacity has no impact on aging, whereas in other models, impaired mitochondrial function can accelerate aging in an ROS-independent fashion.

Although the evidence for ROS contributing to organismal aging is therefore mixed, there is a growing body of work suggesting that oxidants might regulate age-related regenerative capacity by being an important determinant of stem cell biology. Perhaps the first description of this phenomenon came from the analysis briefly mentioned in the preceding section involving mice deficient in the ATM kinase. These mice were known to develop a high rate of tumors; however, it was observed that mice that are tumor free develop an age-dependent decline in hematopoietic function. This defect turned out to be the result in an accelerated decline in self-renewal capacity for the ATM-deficient hematopoietic stem cell (HSC).

Self-renewal is a unique property of stem cells wherein a stem cell can divide and give rise to a daughter stem cell. This property is essential for the maintenance of the overall stem cell pool. Before the observed failure of ATM-deficient HSCs, it was noted that these cells had high levels of ROS.

Indeed, treatment with an antioxidant rescued the self-renewal defect observed in this model. The link between high levels of ROS and stem cell defects was extended by examining the HSC derived from mice that were deficient in three members of the FoxO family of transcription factors. Again, as previously mentioned, the activity of the FoxO family is sensitive to intracellular oxidants, and in turn, FoxO transcription factors can specifically induce the expression of key intracellular antioxidants. HSCs lacking FoxOI, FoxO3, and FoxO4 had reduced expression of antioxidant proteins such as superoxide dismutase and catalase and corresponding increase in ROS levels within the HSC compartment.

As observed with Atm$^{-/-}$ HSCs, FoxO-deficient HSCs demonstrated a marked impairment in self-renewal that could be corrected by antioxidant administration. Similar findings were observed in 2009 by Paik et. and Renault et al. FoxO-deficient neural stem cells.

Finally, mice deficient in the polycomb repressor BmiI also exhibit a defect in self-renewal and a corresponding rise in ROS levels. Taken together, these studies suggest that the age-dependent maintenance of the stem cell pool is intricately connected to regulation of the intracellular redox state. It is tempting to speculate that an age-dependent rise in ROS might contribute to the observed age-dependent decline in stem cell function. However, as we have learned from the previous examples the relationship between a rise in oxidants and the observed pathology is often complex. Echoing this notion, at least in *Drosophila*, oxidants play an essential role in the normal differentiation of HSCs into mature progeny.

Conclusions

Although not exhaustive, the examples discussed highlight the emerging and rapidly expanding role of redox signaling in biology. These studies have implicated the unique chemistry of reactive cysteine residues within certain target proteins. Such redox reactions allows for the covalent modification of protein function in a fashion not unlike the well-established phosphorylation of serine, threonine, and tyrosine residues.

Significant challenges in the field exist, however, including a more precise understanding of how signaling specificity occurs. Often, oxidants are implicated in events in which the levels of ROS may change but where their precise function is inferred and not proven.

This is particularly true in disease states where a rise in oxidants is sometimes **taken as a causal rather than a correlative event.** Progress is also hampered by technical limitations in providing high-throughput means to identify the modification of reactive cysteine residues, as well as accurate and quantitative means of measuring intracellular ROS levels. Newer approaches to address the latter deficiency appear, however, to hold promise.

Over a century has passed since a young Otto Warburg measured the rapid burst of oxygen consumption that occurs as life begins. **Few scientists in his or subsequent generations would have contemplated that at the moment of conception, a fertilized zygote would purposely make prodigious amounts of hydrogen peroxide.**

RMH Note: I believe that the fact that the zygote produces a hydrgen peroxide spike at conception, speaks volumes about the importance of EMODs in reproduction.

Nonetheless, the last two decades have convincingly demonstrated that oxidants can be regulated in their production and specific in their effects. Furthermore, the fact that bacteria and plants also heavily rely on aspects of oxidant signaling suggests that many of these mechanisms are ancient and evolutionarily conserved. A further understanding of these pathways promises to reveal to us many more secrets regarding how life begins, why it ends, and all the myriad complexities that make up the middle.

(Finkel, 2011) http://jcb.rupress.org/content/194/1/7.full

CHAPTER FOURTEEN

PENILE FUNCTION

Penile erection and EMODs

Penile erection is dependent upon vascular smooth muscle relaxation in erectile tissue and penile arteries, the principal mediator of relaxation being nitric oxide (NO). Increased inactivation of NO by superoxide results in impaired penile NO transmission and smooth muscle relaxation. Furthermore, propagation of endothelial dysfunction by ROS may result in chronic impairment of penile vascular function, a process analogous to early atherogenesis. Indeed, ED and atherosclerosis are closely linked through shared risk factors.

Cardiovascular risk factors, erection disorders and endothelium dysfunction

Upon sexual stimulation, penile erection, occurring in response to the activation of pro-erectile autonomic pathways, is greatly dependent on adequate inflow of blood to the erectile tissue and requires coordinated arterial endothelium-dependent vasodilatation and sinusoidal endothelium-dependent corporal smooth muscle relaxation. Nitric oxide (NO) is the principal peripheral pro-erectile neurotransmitter which is released by both non-adrenergic, non-cholinergic neurons and the sinusoidal endothelium to relax corporal smooth muscle through the cGMP pathway.

Any factors modifying the basal corporal tone, the arterial inflow of blood to the corpora, the synthesis/release of neurogenic or endothelial NO are prime suspects for being involved in the pathophysiology of erectile dysfunction (ED). In fact, conditions associated with altered endothelial function, such as ageing, hypertension, hypercholesterolemia and diabetes, may, by changing the balance between contractant and relaxant factors, cause circulatory and structural changes in penile tissues, resulting in arterial insufficiency and defect in smooth muscle relaxation and thus, ED. There is increasing evidence to suggest that ED is predominantly a vascular disease and may even be a marker for occult cardiovascular disease. (Behr-Roussel, 2004)

Hypoxic relaxation of penile arteries: involvement of endothelial nitric oxide and modulation by reactive oxygen species

Although obesity-related cardiovascular disease and hypoxia are associated with erectile dysfunction, little is known about the direct effects of hypoxia on penile arteries. In the present study, the effects of acute hypoxia (Po(2) = approximately 10 Torr, 20 min) were investigated in isolated penile arteries to determine the influence of endothelium removal, nitric oxide (NO) synthase (NOS), cyclooxygenase (COX), NADPH oxidase, changes in reactive oxygen species (ROS), and a high-fat diet. Hypoxia-relaxed penile arteries contracted with phenylephrine by approximately 50%. Relaxation to hypoxia and acetylcholine was reduced by endothelium removal and by inhibition of NOS (N(omega)-nitro-l-arginine) and COX (indomethacin) but was enhanced by Tempol and by NADPH oxidase inhibition with apocynin and gp91ds-tat. Basal superoxide levels detected by lucigenin chemiluminescence were reduced by Tempol and gp91ds-tat and were enhanced by NOS blockade. Hypoxic relaxant responses were enhanced by catalase and ebselen. **Exogenous peroxide evoked relaxations of penile arteries**, which were partially inhibited by endothelium removal and by the inhibition of COX and extracellular signal-regulated mitogen-activated protein kinase (MAPK) but enhanced by p38 MAPK blockade. The NO-dependent component of relaxation to hypoxia was impaired in penile arteries from high-fat diet-fed, obese rats associated with increased superoxide production. Thus hypoxic relaxation of penile arteries is partially mediated by endothelial NO in a manner that is normally attenuated by endogenous ROS production. Obesity further increases superoxide production and impairs the influence of NO. Therefore, cardiovascular disease involving decreased NO bioavailability and/or enhanced ROS generation may contribute to erectile dysfunction through impairing the relaxation of penile arteries to hypoxia. (Prieto et al, 2010)

Penile erection occurs when nitric oxide (NO) released from nerve terminals upon sexual stimulation decreases vascular resistance and increases blood flow through cavernous and helicine arteries, thus stimulating further NO release from penile endothelium, relaxation of corporal smooth muscle, and sustained erection. The enzyme responsible for NO generation NO synthase (NOS) uses l-arginine as a substrate and promotes its oxidation with NADPH and O_2 consumption to yield citrulline and NO. Since molecular O_2 is a substrate for the synthesis of both neural and endothelial NO by NOS, partial O_2 pressure (Po_2) in the blood of the corpus cavernosum plays a key role in the regulation of penile hemodynamics. During the flaccid state, Po_2 is similar to that of venous blood and it rises to 90–100 mmHg during erection as a result of the increased arterial inflow to the sinuses.

Early studies by Kim et al. demonstrated that Po_2 modulates penile erection by regulating NO synthesis in corpus cavernosum tissue and the ability of cavernosal smooth muscle to relax in response to electrical stimulation of the nerves. In addition, responses to endothelium-dependent vasodilators are progressively inhibited as a function of decreasing Po_2 levels. Thus increased blood flow and Po_2 to the penis after arterial dilatation would trigger NO synthesis, relaxation of trabecular smooth muscle, and erection. (Kim et al, 1993)

The effects of chronic hypoxia on erectile function have been reported in both clinical and experimental studies. Erectile dysfunction (ED) is commonly found in male patients with several pathological conditions related with chronic hypoxia such as aging, heart and respiratory failure, sleep apneas, chronic obstructive respiratory disease, diabetes, hypertension, and arteriosclerosis. In a rabbit model of atherosclerosis-induced chronic cavernosal ischemia, both neuronal NOS and endothelial NOS (eNOS) proteins dramatically decrease in erectile tissue, which suggests that arterial insufficiency and subsequent exposure of erectile tissue to hypoxia impair constitutive NOS expression and thus NO synthesis and relaxation. This probably contributes to the arteriogenic ED induced by atherosclerosis and other arterial occlusive diseases.

ED is currently considered as an early sign of subclinical vascular disease and frequently coexists with vascular diseases such as hypertension, atherosclerosis, and diabetes mellitus. Endothelial dysfunction, increased oxidative stress, and reduced NO bioavailability endanger tissue blood flow under these pathological conditions. Studies in prediabetic animal models have demonstrated that hypoxic dilatation of systemic small arteries is impaired because of the scavenging of endothelial mediators by the enhanced generation of reactive oxygen species (ROS) in the arterial wall. (Bagi et al, 2003)

It is well established that the dysregulation of ROS production is involved in the pathogenesis of vascular diseases such as hypertension, hypercholestero- lemia, and diabetes. However, changes in ROS production and in redox status have been hypothesized also to play a role in the O_2 sensing mechanisms of vascular smooth muscle cells. (Wolin, 2009)

Although the association of chronic hypoxia and ED is well documented, the mechanisms underlying the acute effects of hypoxia on the integrated function of erectile tissue are not well understood. (Kim et al, 1996). Most systemic blood vessels relax to hypoxia as a part of local autoregulatory mechanisms that match blood perfusion to the metabolic demands of the tissue.

Effect of scavenging peroxide with catalase or ebselen on hypoxia- and ACh-induced relaxation.

To assess an influence of endogenous peroxide on the hypoxic relaxant responses of penile arteries, the effects of catalase and ebselen were tested. Scavenging peroxide with catalase (200 U/ml) markedly enhanced hypoxia- and ACh-induced relaxations. Ebselen, a glutathione peroxidase mimetic that can decrease intracellular peroxide (Gao et al, 2009), induced an even greater enhancement of the hypoxic and ACh relaxant responses in penile arteries.

Effect of exogenous H_2O_2 on penile arteries.

An exogenous addition of H_2O_2 (1–100 µM) caused a concentration-depend- ent relaxation of Phe-precontracted penile arteries, with the maximum response at 100 µM being 85 ± 3% ($n = 16$). A biphasic response consisting of a transient contraction followed by a profound and persistent relaxation was often observed at the highest concentrations of H_2O_2. Scavenging per- oxide with catalase (200 U/ml) blunted relaxation to exogenous H_2O_2. The removal of the endothelium reduced the contractile component of the response to H_2O_2 at the highest concentration used (100 µM) to 54 ± 9% ($P < 0.01$ vs. control, $n = 6$). The inhibition of cyclooxygenase with indomethacin (1 µM) blunted the relaxations elicited by low concentrations of H_2O_2. Since the vascular effects of peroxide can be mediated through the activation of both the ERK MAPK and the p38 MAPK, the effects of selective inhibitors were assessed on the exogenous peroxide-elicited relaxations. PD-98050 (10 µM) inhibited the relaxation responses elicited by low concentrations of H_2O_2, suggesting that ERK MAPK influenced the observed relaxation responses. In contrast, SB-203580 (10 μM) enhanced the H_2O_2-elicited relaxation, suggesting that p38 MAPK has a negative modulatory effect upon peroxide-induced relaxation in penile arteries.

The effects of dietary fat-induced obesity on the relaxant responses to hypoxia are shown and on the basal superoxide production of penile arteries. The relaxation induced by acute hypoxia was significantly impaired in arteries from HFD-fed animals, whereas the contractile responses upon reoxygenation were unchanged compared with control arteries. **A quantification of superoxide production in intact arteries by lucigenin-enhanced chemiluminescence demonstrated that basal superoxide production was significantly enhanced by about twofold in arteries of high fat diet (HFD) rats.** (Erdei et al, 2006)

To determine whether impaired synthesis/release of NO is involved in the impaired relaxation of penile arteries to hypoxia, the effect of inhibition of NO synthesis was assessed.

Penile arteries responded to acute hypoxia with a significant relaxation similar to that found in other systemic arteries and also in penile corpus cavernosum, where hypoxia induced relaxation and the accumulation of intracellular Ca^{2+}. (Kim et al, 1996)

Although a significant fraction of the penile hypoxic relaxant response originates from vascular smooth muscle, the present results demonstrate that the endothelium modulates this response, and endothelium-derived mediators including both NO and relaxant prostanoids appear to be involved in the relaxation to acute hypoxia that is observed. These data are consistent with earlier observations in other systemic arteries such as skeletal muscle and coronary small arteries from the rat. However, the mechanisms for relaxation to hypoxia in penile arteries seem to differ from those in penile corpus cavernosum, because the response in this tissue was found to be independent of the endothelium, suggesting differences in the signaling pathways that control relaxation of penile erectile tissues under hypoxic conditions. (Kim et al, 1996)

The participation of ROS in the vascular O_2 sensing mechanisms remains a matter of debate. (Wolin, 2009), and both ROS generated by either Nox or mitochondria (Michelakis et al, 2002) and ROS-independent pathways have been suggested to play a role in the arterial responses to hypoxia.

An exposure to acute hypoxia significantly decreased basal superoxide levels measured by lucigenin chemiluminescence in intact penile arteries, which recovered to control levels upon reoxygenation. The enhancing effect of ROS scavengers on the relaxation to hypoxia despite the inhibitory effect of hypoxia on superoxide production could be explained on the basis of the interactions between basally released superoxide and NO released by hypoxia. Thus a significant basal production of superoxide increased by PKC activation and blunted by Tempol was found in penile arteries. Vascular smooth muscle from resistance arteries contains Nox2, a Nox also known as gp91^{phox}. The modest inhibitory effect of Nox2 inhibition on basal superoxide production suggests that other sources also contribute to ROS production in penile arteries. This is consistent with findings in systemic arteries from Nox2-deficient mice where superoxide production was unaltered by Nox2 deletion. (Miller et al, 2009)

Also, **in human vessels, superoxide production by the Nox system was greater in veins than arteries, where other sources such as xanthine oxidase substantially contribute to superoxide production.** (Guzik et al, 2004) (Guzik TJ, Sadowski J, Kapelak B, Jopek A, Rudzinski P, Pillai R, Korbut R, Channon KM. Systemic regulation of vascular NAD(P)H oxidase activity and nox isoform expression in human arteries and veins. *Arterioscler Thromb Vasc Biol* 24: 1614–1620, 2004) (Guzik et al, 2002)

Thus ROS can modulate hypoxia-induced vasodilatation by decreasing NO bioavailability through quenching by superoxide in a manner that is associated with the formation of peroxynitrite.

Hypoxia and the inhibition of the electron transport chain increases mitochondrial ROS generation in arterial smooth muscle, and the subsequent dismutation of superoxide to peroxide makes ROS readily diffusible across mitochondrial membranes. (Gao et al, 2009) (Michelakis et al, 2002)

Several earlier studies have shown impaired hypoxic vasodilator responses in arteries from animal models of cardiovascular disease. Obesity, along with a constellation of metabolic and vascular abnormalities including insulin resistance, dyslipidemia and hypertension, jointly referred to as metabolic syndrome, markedly increases the risk for cardiovascular disease and diabetes. These metabolic alterations are associated with endothelial dysfunction, and they act as independent risk factors for ED.

The present findings therefore suggest that enhanced ROS production is probably interfering with the NO signaling of penile arteries, thus impairing NO-mediated hypoxic relaxant responses.

In summary, the present study provides evidence for the involvement of endothelial-derived NO and its modulation by ROS in the hypoxic relaxation of penile arteries. Decreased NO bioavailability and enhanced ROS production impair penile hypoxic responses and contribute to the endothelial/vascular dysfunction in dietary fat-induced obesity.

It seems to me that weight reduction, avoidance of high fat diets, increasing oxygen consumption all improve sexual performance, even though they increase EMOD production.

Sex hormone suppression and sexual impotence in hypoxic pulmonary fibrosis Eight men with hypoxia associated with idiopathic pulmonary fibrosis were studied. Serum testosterone concentrations were low in two subjects and fell to subnormal levels in two others as the clinical condition and arterial oxygen tension deteriorated. There was a significant correlation between serum testosterone concentrations and arterial oxygen tensions (p less than 0.05). Three patients showed evidence of suppression of luteinising hormone secretion at the pituitary level. Only occasional abnormalities of thyroid and prolactin concentrations were noted. Most of the men suffered from organic sexual impotence, which is considered to be due at least in part to endocrine disturbance. These findings are similar to observations in patients with hypoxic chronic obstructive airways disease and support the hypothesis that hypoxia of lung disease suppresses the hypothalamo-pituitary-testicular axis. (Semple et al, 1984)

Reversal of sexual impotence in male patients with chronic obstructive pulmonary disease and hypoxemia with long-term oxygen therapy

Erectile impotence is commonly encountered in male patients with respiratory failure and hypoxia. In this study, 42% of the patients experienced reversal of sexual impotence during long-term oxygen therapy (LTOT). We examine the association between sexual impotence, gonadal axis hormones, hypoxia, and oxygen therapy. Nineteen sexually impotent male patients eligible for LTOT (pO2 < 7.3 kPa during stable disease) and with sexual impotence received oxygen therapy for 1 month (n = 12) or 24 h (n = 7). pO2, LH, FSH, testosterone, and SHBG (sex hormone binding globulin) were monitored. **Five of 12 patients receiving oxygen for 1 month regained sexual potency. The responders showed a significant increase in arterial pO2 and serum testosterone, and a decline in SHBG compared to non-responders.** None of the patients receiving oxygen for 24 h experienced reversal of sexual impotence, despite a significant increase in pO2. In these patients, serum testosterone did not increase significantly. **Reversal of sexual impotence may be achieved in some patients with respiratory failure.** The oxygen therapy must, however be administered for an adequate length of time. (Aasebo et al, 1993)

Dietary antioxidants improve arteriogenic erectile dysfunction

Most cases of erectile dysfunction (ED) are associated with oxidative stress risk factors such as diabetes mellitus, smoking, hypercholesterolemia and hypertension. Our goal was to search for markers of oxidative stress in arteriogenic ED and examine the protective role of dietary antioxidants. Atherosclerosis-induced ED was developed in rabbits by balloon de-endothelialization of the iliac arteries. Ballooned and age-matched control animals were assigned into subgroups receiving pomegranate extract antioxidants in drinking water or tap water as placebo. After 8 weeks, penile blood flow and erectile activity were recorded. Erectile tissue relaxation, oxidative products, oxidative stress-responsive genes and structure were examined using organ bath, enzyme immunoassay, quantitative real-time polymerase chain reaction and transmission electron microscopy, respectively. Arterial ballooning caused diffused atherosclerosis, decreased intracavernosal blood flow and led to ED. Impairment of endothelium-dependent relaxation, diffused fibrosis, increased oxidative products, upregulation of superoxide dismutase (SOD) and aldose reductase (AR) gene expression, mitochondrial and endothelial structural damage and increased caveolae were evident in erectile tissues from atherosclerotic animals receiving placebo. **Upregulation of antioxidant enzymes SOD and AR failed to protect ischemic erectile tissue from oxidative injury. Pomegranate extract significantly improved intracavernosal blood flow, erectile activity, smooth muscle relaxation and fibrosis of the atherosclerotic group in comparison with the atherosclerotic group receiving placebo, but did not normalize them to the age-matched control levels.** Pomegranate extract appeared more effective in diminishing oxidative products, preventing SOD and AR gene upregulation, and protecting mitochondrial, endothelial and caveolae structural integrity of the atherosclerotic group. Our data suggest the presence of oxidative stress in ED and a more efficient action of antioxidants on molecular and ultrastructural alterations than on distinct functional deficit and structural damage in the ischemic penis. (Zhang et al, 2011)

CHAPTER FIFTEEN

Alleged EMOD damage

For review purposes, I need to repeat the alleged damages caused by EMODs.

Allegedly, EMODs (oxidative stress) have been hypothesized to cause the following damage:

- damage of the sperm plasma membrane
- cause a loss of DNA integrity
- lead to a failure of conception
- cause miscarriages
- cause spontaneous abortions
- cause idiopathic recurrent pregnancy loss
- cause hydatidiform mole
- cause defective embryogenesis
- cause drug-induced teratogenicity
- cause oxidant-induced endothelial damage, impaired placental vascularization and immune malfunction
- cause multifactorial and polygenic etiologies of abortion, recurrent pregnancy loss and defective embryogenesis
- cause intrauterine growth restriction and fetal dysmorphogenesis
- oxidant stress has been linked to the formation of antiphospholipid antibodies in the antiphospholipid syndrome
- may even cause childhood cancer
- cause male infertility
- cause sperm dysfunction
- reduce male reproductive potential

- cause endometriosis, ovarian cancer, and polycystic ovary disease via proinflammatory cytokines
- male and female infertility, including fetal dysmorphogenesis, abortions, and intrauterine growth restriction
- damage spermatogenesis and Leydig cell steroidogenesis
- cause erectile dysfunction (ED)
- and finally, (and allegedly), peroxidative damage is currently regarded as the single most important cause of impaired testicular function underpinning the pathological consequences of a wide range of conditions from testicular torsion to diabetes and xenobiotic exposure.

Testes, radicals and antioxidants

In order to address this risk, the testes have developed a sophisticated array of antioxidant systems comprising both enzymatic and non-enzymatic constituents. (Aitken, Roman, 2008)

Spermatogenesis is an extremely active replicative process capable of generating approximately 1,000 sperm a second. The high rates of cell division inherent in this process imply correspondingly high rates of mitochondrial oxygen consumption by the germinal epithelium. However, the poor vascularization of the testes means that oxygen tensions in this tissue are low and that competition for this vital element within the testes is extremely intense.

According to Aitken and Roman, despite the low oxygen tensions that characterize the testicular micro-environment, this tissue remains vulnerable to oxidative stress due to the abundance of highly unsaturated fatty acids (particularly 20:4 and 22:6) and the presence of potential reactive oxygen species (ROS)-generating systems.

EMOD generation can be from the mitochondria and a variety of enzymes including the xanthine- and NADPH-oxidases, and the cytochrome P450s. These enzymes specialize in the professional generation of EMODs or produce these toxic metabolites as an inadvertent consequence of their biochemical activity.

In order to address this risk, the testes have developed a sophisticated array of antioxidant systems comprising both enzymatic and non-enzymatic constituents. Concerning the enzymatic constituents of this defense system, **the induction of oxidative stress in the testes precipitates a response characterized by the NFκB mediated induction of mRNA species for superoxide dismutase (SOD), glutathione peroxidase (GPx) and glutathione-S-transferase (GST) activities.**

The fundamental biochemistry of these antioxidant enzymes involves **the rapid conversion of superoxide anion (O_2^-) to hydrogen peroxide (H_2O_2) in the presence of SOD in order to prevent the former from participating in the formation of highly pernicious hydroxyl radicals.** The H_2O_2 generated in this manner is a **powerful membrane permeant oxidant** in its own right **that has to be rapidly eliminated from the cell in order to prevent the induction of oxidative damage to lipids, proteins and DNA.**

The elimination of H_2O_2 is either effected by catalase or **glutathione peroxidase, with the latter predominating in the case of the testes.** GST on the other hand involves a large and complex family of proteins that catalyze the conjugation of reduced glutathione via the sulfhydryl group to electrophilic centers on a wide variety of substrates in preparation for excretion from the cell. This activity is critical in the detoxification of peroxidized lipids as well as the metabolism of xenobiotics.

Given the importance of SOD in this defense strategy, it is not surprising that the testes contain not only the conventional cytosolic (Cu/Zn) and mitochondrial (Fe/Mn) forms of SOD but also feature **an unusual form of extracellular SOD, (SOD-Ex) which is produced by both Sertoli and germ cells, particularly the former.**

The importance of the cytosolic form of SOD (SOD1) was recently emphasized in studies of **SOD1-knockout mice subjected to testicular heat stress.** This treatment induced significantly enhanced levels of DNA strand breakage and cytochrome C leakage from the mitochondria of germ cells in these animals compared with the wild-type controls.

I believe that the absence of SOD leads to an EMOD insufficiency (H_2O_2), which in turn, leads to the DNA damage.

Similarly, the importance of **the mitochondrial form of SOD (SOD2) in controlling O_2^- leakage from testicular mitochondria has been emphasized by the finding that the mRNA for this enzyme is markedly higher in the testes** than the liver, unlike GPx and catalase. Moreover, SOD-2 mRNA levels are developmentally and translationally regulated with maximal levels of expression in early post-meiotic germ cells.

Although **catalase is of limited importance in the testes**, there are several isoforms of GPx in this tissue that use glutathione (GSH) as a source of electrons to reduce H_2O_2 to water. They are concentrated in the mitochondria, nucleus and acrosomal domain of differentiating spermatozoa. The phospholipid hydroperoxide GPx (PHGPx) is one of the most important GPx isoforms in a testicular context and is highly expressed in both spermatogenic and Leydig cells.

Since most forms of GPx are selenium dependent it is possible to gauge the importance of these enzymes in the support of testicular function by examining the impact of selenium deficiency on male reproduction. **Animals fed on a selenium deficient diet exhibit a significant reduction of testicular GPx activity and an accompanying loss of germ cells from the germinal epithelium of the testes.** Moreover, selenium administration prior to the creation of oxidative stress in the testes using the torsion/detorsion model to create ischemia-reperfusion injury, has been found to suppress lipid peroxidation and improve the histopathological profile. **I believe that this is compounded by the fact that elemental selenium is a prooxidant.**

Also, we must keep in mind that peroxide is a substrate for the GPx enzymes and the purpose of these enzymes is not to "destroy" peroxide because they need it to accomplish their enzymatic function.

Reportedly, the testes rely heavily on small molecular weight antioxidant factors for protection against oxidative damage.

Zinc

Zinc is an acknowledged antioxidant factor that as well as being a core constituent of free radical scavenging enzymes such as SOD and **a recognized protector of sulfhydryl groups**, is also thought to impair lipid peroxidation by displacing transition metals such as iron and copper from catalytic sites. Rats fed a zinc deficient diet experience a decrease in testicular antioxidant potential and a concomitant increase of lipid peroxidation in this tissue. Conversely, zinc administration will counteract the oxidative stress created in the testes by exposure to lead.

However, zinc can have both prooxidant and anti-oxidant activity, which also complicates the interpretation of this data. Among the essential trace metals, zinc has the greatest number and variety of functions in hundreds of enzymes and thousands of protein domains with different types of zinc finger motifs. In spite of the fact that zinc ions are redox-inert in biology, they have profound effects on redox metabolism. Thus, both zinc deficiency and zinc overload elicit oxidative stress that can lead to the death of nerve cells (and likely other cell types). These pro-oxidant functions contrast with pro-antioxidant functions in a range of physiological zinc concentrations. (Hao and Maret, 2005)

Vitamin E and C

It has been recognized since the 1940s that **vitamin E (alpha-tocopherol) is a powerful lipophilic antioxidant that is absolutely vital for the maintenance of mammalian spermatogenesis.** However, there is little or no discussion of overloading with either of these vitamins.

Vitamin C (ascorbic acid) also contributes to the support of spermatogenesis at least in part through its capacity to reduce alpha-tocopherol **and maintain this antioxidant in an active state.** Vitamin C is itself maintained in a reduced state by a GSH-dependent dehydroascorbate reductase, which is abundant in the testes. **Deficiencies of vitamins C or E leads to a state of oxidative stress in the testes that disrupts both spermatogenesis and the production of testosterone.**

Conversely, ascorbate administration to normal animals stimulates both sperm production and testosterone secretion. This vitamin also counteracts the testicular oxidative stress induced by exposure to pro-oxidants such as arsenic, PCBs (Arochlor 1254), cadmium, endosulfan and alcohol.

Furthermore, endogenous ascorbate levels decrease dramatically when oxidative stress is induced in the testes by, for example, chronic exposure to lead, chromium, cadmium or aflatoxin. Vitamin E has also been shown to suppress lipid peroxidation in testicular microsomes and mitochondria and to reverse the detrimental effects of oxidative stress on testicular function mediated by exposure to such factors as ozone, iron overload, intensive exercise or exposure to aflatoxin, PCB, cyclophosphamide formaldehyde.

Another small molecular mass free radical scavenger that has recently been shown to play a major role in reducing H_2O_2 is a testes-specific form of cytochrome C. This cytochrome C isoform is also a powerful activator of apoptosis, providing additional protection to the testes by virtue of its ability to facilitate the depletion of damaged germ cells. It can also be said that H_2O_2 also induces apoptosis.

The pineal hormone melatonin (N-acetyl, 5-methoxytryptamine) also plays a major role in protecting the testes from oxidative stress, given the significant stimulatory effect of pinealectomy on the oxidative damage recorded in the testes as a consequence of induced hyperthyroidism. Melatonin has two major attributes that set it apart from most other antioxidants. Firstly, it undergoes a two electron oxidation when acting as antioxidant, rather than the one electron oxidation favored by many free radical scavengers. As a result, this compound cannot redox cycle and inadvertently generate free radicals.

Cryptorchidism

The elevated temperatures associated with experimental cryptorchidism are associated with oxidative stress in the testes and a reduction in SOD and catalase activities. Consistent with these findings, direct exposure of spermatogenic cells to elevated temperatures was found to induce high rates of apoptosis via mechanisms that were associated with elevated levels of H_2O_2 generation and could be ameliorated by the addition of catalase.

Moreover, the consequence of heat stress on spermatogenic cells was exacerbated in SOD1-knock out mice via mechanisms that could be reversed by the addition of Tiron, a superoxide anion radical scavenger. The clinical significance of this finding can be seen in the high levels of DNA damage and ROS generation seen in the spermatozoa of patients with a history of cryptorchidism.

Testicular torsion

Prolonged torsion leads to testicular ischemia and high levels of oxidative stress in the ipsilateral testes associated with NO and H_2O_2 production, increased lipid peroxide formation, isoprostane accumulation, antioxidant enzyme depletion and increased rates of mitochondria-mediated apoptosis in the germ line.

Significantly, the level of peroxidative damage observed in testicular tissue increases following detorsion, indicating the induction of reperfusion injury. The tissue injury induced by testicular torsion/detorsion can be dramatically alleviated by pretreatment with exogenous antioxidants such as selenium, resveratrol, L-carnitine, caffeic acid phenethyl ester and garlic extract.

In animal models prolonged testicular torsion results in excessive ROS generation, depletion of antioxidant enzymes and the appearance of oxidative damage in the contralateral testes. In light of these data, surgical removal of the ipsilateral testes would seem warranted if the period of ischemia has been extensive.

Varicocele

The impaired venous drainage to the testes seen with varicocele is also associated with the disruption of spermatogenesis via mechanisms involving the induction of oxidative stress. In a recent study, surgical correction of left sided varicocele was shown to significantly improve sperm concentration, total count, morphology and motility in concert with significant improvements in the antioxidant status of the spermatozoa and seminal plasma. The general concept that testicular pathologies associated with varicocele are linked with the induction of oxidative stress has been confirmed in animal models. The pathological consequences of experimental varicocele induction can be significantly reversed by the concomitant administration of an antioxidant, melatonin.

The site of free radical generation in varicocele patients is still open to conjecture.

On the one hand, enhanced free radical generation by the spermatozoa and/ or precursor germ cells has been repeatedly suggested, on the other, there is evidence to suggest that excess free radical generation may involve the spermatic vein itself.

The presence of excess cytoplasm has been positively correlated with the generation of ROS by human spermatozoa, via mechanisms involving the facilitated supply NADPH to oxidases in the sperm plasma membrane. These enzymes, including NOX5 and DUOX, both of which have been identified in human spermatozoa, are normally deprived of sufficient NADPH to drive free radical generation; what hexose monophosphate shunt activity there is, being largely devoted to the maintenance of glutathione reductase activity.

Hyperthyroidism

The induction of hyperthyroidism in rats is associated with oxidative stress in the testes as reflected by increased lipid peroxidation, elevated GSH levels and induction of antioxidant enzymes. The oxidative stress appears to be associated with a thyroxine dependent increase in mitochondrial activity and concomitant leakage of electrons from the mitochondrial electron transport chain. **Hypothyroidism can induce oxidative stress in the testes as reflected by enhanced levels of H_2O_2 production and increased carbonyl generation.**

I can also interpret most of this data as indicating that the increase in antioxidant enzymes triggers the release of more EMODs, with the excessive antioxidant enzyme levels as being causative of the damaging effects seen. Which came first?

Diabetes

Experimental induction of diabetes in animal models has been shown to impair testicular function and decrease male fertility. Thus, diabetogens such as streptozotocin, enhance ROS generation and induce both lipid peroxidation and protein carbonyl expression in the testes. **In light of recent data showing an increased level of DNA damage in the spermatozoa of diabetic patients compared with non-diabetic controls, causative links between diabetes, oxidative stress in the male germ line and DNA damage appears both likely and clinically, extremely important.**

Yet, they do not address the fact that hyperglycemia can suppress EMOD levels.

Infection

Experimental models of infection, involving the intraperitoneal injection of bacterial lipopolysaccharide (LPS), induced lipid peroxidation in the testes and rapidly depleted this tissue of antioxidant enzyme activity in the form of SOD, catalase and the glutathione peroxidase-reductase couple. This oxidative stress was associated with the transient generation of pro-inflammatory mediators such as interleukin Iβ, inducible nitric oxide synthase and cyclo-oxygenase-2.

I believe that the reduction in antioxidant enzymes is necessary for the body to mobilize an adequate EMOD defense against the infective agent.

Exercise

Excess exercise can cause oxidative stress in the testes and generate high levels of lipid peroxidation in association with significant declines in the activities of key antioxidant enzymes including SOD, catalase, GST and GPx. Please remember that exercise is good for us!! (Manna, Samanta, 2003)

The endocrine environment

Treatments including exposure to cyclophosphamide or dimethane sulfonate that diminish the intratesticular concentration of testosterone, inhibit the testicular expression of antioxidant enzymes such as GPx, SOD and catalase.

Intriguingly, the suppression of antioxidant activity in response to **exogenous steroid treatment** largely affects the Leydig cells that contain most of the catalase and GPx activities.

Interestingly, **over-stimulation of the Leydig cells by chronic exposure to hCG (100 IU/day for 30 days in rats) also stimulates high levels of ROS production from these germ cells**, that in turn stimulate lipid peroxidation, reduction in antioxidant enzyme activities, germ cell apoptosis and the consequential disruption of spermatogenesis.

A stable redox environment depends on an appropriately balanced system.

Retinoids

The Sertoli cell has been shown to generate EMODs following stimulation with all trans-retinoic acid (RA), a vital cofactor for spermatogenesis. There may be nothing particularly specific about this effect since **retinoids have been shown to stimulate ROS generation in a variety of other cellular systems.**

Nevertheless, **the free radical generation triggered by retinoids in the testes may explain the testicular degeneration induced by hypervitaminosis A in the rat and the association between excess beta carotene intake and infertility in human males.** (Biswas, Deb, 1965)

Xenobiotics

A wide variety of **xenobiotics have been shown to induce oxidative stress in the testes** in concert with the suppression of antioxidant mechanisms and a summary of these **testicular toxicants** follows:

Smoking; alcohol; chromic acid; iron; lead; cadmium; uranium; arsenic; vanadate; phthalate esters; sulfur dioxide; sodium fluoride; PCB/PCN; Metoxychlor: bisphenol A; nonylphenol: adreamycin; cisplatin; cyclophosphamide; hexachlorocyclohexane; trinitroluene; aflatoxin; lindane; quinalphos; endosulfan; diethyl maleate; monensin; formaldehyde; alloxan; streptozotocin; acrylamide; ozone. (Aitken, Roman, 2008)

Oxidant toxicants

Thus, any of these "oxidant-toxicants" could be used to increase oxidative capacity of the body. Chromium, for example, is a testicular toxicant that stimulates lipid peroxidation and suppresses antioxidant enzyme activities as well as ascorbate levels in the testes.

Studies in monkeys have also shown that chromium administration decreases not only inhibit the classical array of antioxidant enzymes in the testes but also diminishes the testicular content of GSH as well as vitamins A,E and C, while H_2O_2 production and hydroxyl radical formation are increased. Additional transition metals such as iron also induce lipid peroxidation, protein carbonyl expression and lipid soluble antioxidant depletion in testicular tissue with the consequent disruption of spermatogenesis.

Heavy metals

Heavy metals such as lead, cadmium and uranium have a similar effect on the testes disrupting spermatogenesis via mechanisms that involved the induction of lipid peroxidation, depletion of ROS scavengers and disruption of testicular antioxidant enzyme activity. Similarly, **vanadate is a testicular toxicant that induces lipid peroxidation in the testes** along with significant suppression of testicular SOD and catalase and the disruption of 3β- and 17β-hydroxysteroid dehydrogenase activities.

Other oxidant toxicants

Here I list a wide variety of different industrial and environmental toxicants that are all capable of compromising male fertility by inducing a state of oxidative stress in the testes. These compounds include;

- phthalate esters,
- sulfur dioxide,
- sodium fluoride,
- a range of environmental estrogens (e.g., PCBs, methoxychlor, bisphenol A nonylphenol),
- chemotherapeutic agents (e.g., adriamycin, cisplatin cyclophosphamide)
- hexachlorocyclohexane,
- 2,4,6-trinitrotoluene,
- aflatoxin,
- lindane,
- quinalphos endosulfan,
- diethyl maleate,
- monensin,
- formaldehyde,
- alloxan,
- streptozotocin,
- acrylamide
- and ozone.

Oxidative stress is also produced by:
- ethanol,
- indomethacin,
- X-irradiation,
- streptozotocin-induced diabetes.

In vitro studies have also shown that melatonin and its immediate precursor N-acetyl-serotonin could inhibit ascorbate-Fe (II) induced lipid peroxidation in rat testicular microsomes and mitochondria. **Is this another indicator that ascorbate can have prooxidant activity?**

Physical factors such as static magnetic fields and electromagnetic radiation in its various forms from heat to X-ray irradiation, can also trigger a state of oxidative stress in testicular tissue.

Antioxidant therapy

The testicular torsion-detorsion model has been repeatedly used to determine the relative potential of different antioxidants.

This model involves the application of antioxidant therapy prior to the creation of a brief period of oxidative stress and subsequent comparison of various testicular attributes (lipid peroxidation, histopathology, DNA damage or antioxidant enzyme status) with sham operated controls (Table 2).

Such analyses have recorded **significant protection against oxidative stress for factors such as:**

- garlic extract,
- caffeic acid phenethyl ester (CAPE),
- N-acetyl cysteine,
- pentoxifylline,
- erdostein,
- resveratrol,
- dexpathenol,
- L-carnitine
- and propofol anesthetic.
(Aitken, Roman, 2008)

A variety of antioxidants have also been assessed for their ability to counteract oxidative stress in the testes created by alternative mechanisms. For example: (1) CAPE has been shown to protect the testes from the oxidative stress created by exposure to **dizocilpine (MK-801)**, a drug that is commonly used to induce schizophrenia, and cigarette smoke (2) **lycopene, the red plant antioxidant that is a major constituent of tomatoes, is capable of reversing the oxidative damage induced in rat testes following exposure to cyclosporin A or cisplatin** (3) extracts from the herb *Lycium barbarum*, effectively protect the testes from the oxidative damage induced by heat stress and significantly suppress the oxidative DNA damage induced in mouse testicular cells by H_2O_2 (4) MTEC (an aqueous-methanol extract of *Musa paradisiaca, Tamarindus indica, Eugenia jambolana* and *Coccinia indica*) protects against the oxidative testicular damage resulting from induced diabetes (5) lecithin administration protects the testes from the oxidative stress induced by chronic ethanol exposure (6) **lipoic acid has been shown to inhibit the oxidative damage resulting from exposure to cyclophosphamide, adriamycin and X-irradiation** (7) complex feruloyl oligosaccharides released from wheat bran have also been shown to protect the testes from the oxidative stress associated with alloxan-induced diabetes in rats and (8) **Beta-carotene** ameliorates cadmium induced oxidative stress in the testes, suppressing lipid peroxidation and restoring SOD, GST and GSH to normal physiological levels.

RMH interpretation of the data and cautions

Here we go again, the evil EMODs are being taken out by the heroic antioxidants. This is the exact same old tired pattern we have seen with cancer, heart disease, stroke, diabetes, arthritis, etc.

For those who believe this nonscience/nonsense, keep in mind the inarguable fact that EMODs are essential for proper cellular function and without them, the cell dies. Antioxidants can interfere with the normal functioning of the cell when they reach excessive levels.

While it is true that we need a certain level of antioxidants for normal cellular functioning, excessive levels will cause us to lose our ability to fight infections and cancer. Antioxidant overload will prevent us from being able to make adequate energy for our daily lives. They will lead to increases in infections, cancer, heart disease, strokes and our overall mortality, according to the evidence-based data.

On the surface, blaming everything bad on EMODs may all look great, in that this wide variety of antioxidants are blocking so-called oxidative stress but keep in mind that **these antioxidants are non-specific inhibitors of all oxidative reactions.**

This includes crucial redox reactions necessary for cell survival and maintenance of homeostasis. Also, as in my book, *Dangers of Excessive Antioxidants In Cancer Patients*, **these antioxidants can be acting against the very intent of therapies such as chemotherapy, photodynamic therapy and radiation therapy, wherein they are shielding the cancer cells.**

This is an extremely important consideration before recommending antioxidants to treat or counter rather harmless or benign conditions. The antioxidants can shield the cancer cells and protect them from being killed by oxidant induced apoptosis.

The concept of the **"oxidant toxicant"** may apply to dead cells in a test tube but it is not applicable to the living/breathing cell. In the living breathing cell, oxidation is one of our most essential chemical reactions and antioxidants can act directly against it, especially if they are present in excessive amounts. We must strive to function in the realm of **"oxidative bliss."**

I believe that we should be discussing **the "anti-oxidant toxicant"** instead!

Moreover, **these in vitro and in vivo studies in animals do not produce the same beneficial results in randomized controlled trials (RCTs) in humans.** There is a huge disconnect between laboratory studies and the RCTs.

Personally, **I believe that all of the antioxidants used above should be used with great caution.** These include:

- garlic extract,
- caffeic acid phenethyl ester (CAPE),
- N-acetyl cysteine,
- pentoxifylline,
- erdostein,
- resveratrol,
- dexpathenol,
- L-carnitine,
- propofol anesthetic,
- lycopene,
- extracts from the herb *Lycium barbarum*, MTEC (an aqueous-methanol extract of *Musa paradisiaca, Tamarindus indica, Eugenia jambolana* and *Coccinia indica*),
- lecithin,
- lipoic acid,
- vitamins A, C & E,
- complex feruloyl oligosaccharides released from wheat bran,
- beta-carotene,
- morphine,
- pentoxyphillene,
- tiron,
- melatonin, etc.

It is said that one of the most effective antioxidants for the protection of testicular function is melatonin.

Antioxidants have frequently been administered to infertile men in the hope of improving the quality of the semen profile. Very few properly controlled double blind crossover trials have been conducted in this context.

Aitken and Roman conclude that, "**Oxidative stress is a major factor in the etiology of male infertility.**" A large number of independent clinical studies have demonstrated a correlative relationship between male infertility and evidence of oxidative stress in the ejaculate. Moreover the literature reviewed in this chapter reveals an abundance of experimental data in animal models demonstrating a causal relationship between the induction of oxidative stress in the testes and the impairment of male reproductive function. **However these two lines of evidence have not yet come together.**

Although oxidative stress is clearly a dominant feature in the etiology of male infertility, **the underlying causative mechanisms remain unresolved.**

That there are so many factors capable of inducing oxidative stress in the testes strongly suggests that **this is a vulnerable tissue that is both highly dependent on oxygen to drive spermatogenesis** and **yet highly susceptible to the toxic effects of reactive oxygen metabolites;** in this context, the **testis is very like the brain.** And the brain can do quite well, while constantly bathed in EMODs, for up to 100 years of age.

Aitken and Roman believe that **there are clear benefits to be gained by treating susceptible individuals with exogenous antioxidants.** Yet, …. little effort has gone into the development of such a preparation and **how poor most of the clinical trials in this area have been. Basically, the clinical trials have been failures.**

For the above section by Aitken and Roman, references should be obtained by referring to their original article: http://www.ncbi.nlm.nih.gov/pmc/articles/PMC2715191/?tool=pubmed

or (Aitken, Roman, 2008)

CHAPTER SIXTEEN

Oxygen free radicals and the penis

Penile erections involve an integration of complex physiologic processes involving the CNS, peripheral nervous system, and hormonal and vascular systems. Any abnormality involving these systems, whether from medication or disease, has a significant impact on the ability to develop and sustain an erection, ejaculate, and experience orgasm. Tumescence, the vascular filling of the cavernous bodies, relies on neural and hormonal mechanisms operating at various levels of the neural axis. This is unique among visceral functions because it requires central neurological input.

Erectile function is best understood in the context of overall male sexual function. This involves distinct phases that include arousal (libido), erection, orgasm, ejaculation, and a refractory period.

One thing is clear. Libido comes from hormones but an erection is produced by free radicals, specifically NO.

Thus, the first question that comes to mind is, **"If erection is strictly dependent upon free radicals, what is the anticipated effect of excessive antioxidants?"** Logically, antioxidant overload would be expected to inhibit or prevent penile erection.

The authors have talked of the wondrous manner in which a wide range of antioxidants have been shown to block the damaging effects of free radicals, but none have addressed the possibility that excessive antioxidant levels will block the necessary and beneficial activities of free radicals. This possibility can not be overlooked any longer. Instead, they talk of nitric oxide being negated by another free radical, superoxide anion. Why are they afraid to address the area of antioxidant overkill?

One must use extreme care when altering antioxidant defenses. The redox balance is a critical aspect of all aerobic life. EMODs are signaling mechanisms for a vast range of vital metabolic pathways and networks, including those involved in sexual performance.

Penile erection is dependent upon vascular smooth muscle relaxation in erectile tissue and penile arteries, the principal mediator of relaxation being nitric oxide (NO). RMH Note: This free radical response can be theoretically blocked by antioxidants.

However, increased inactivation of NO by superoxide results in impaired penile NO transmission and smooth muscle relaxation. Furthermore, propagation of endothelial dysfunction by ROS may result in chronic impairment of penile vascular function, a process analogous to early atherogenesis. Indeed, ED and atherosclerosis are closely linked through shared risk factors. (Jones et al, 2002)

Traditional beta-blockers have sometimes been associated with erectile dysfunction (ED). Nebivolol is a cardioselective beta(1)-adrenoceptor antagonist that promotes vasodilation through a nitric oxide (NO)-dependent mechanism. Nebivolol in vitro potentiated NO/cGMP-mediated relaxation of human erectile tissues. These effects may account for the low incidence of ED in nebivolol-treated hypertensive patients. Nebivolol dilates human penile arteries and reverses erectile dysfunction in diabetic rats through enhancement of nitric oxide signaling. (Angulo et al, 2010)

When blood vessel and cultured endothelial cells from hypertensive animals are treated with nebivolol, there is a decrease in superoxide production and an increase in the expression and activity of endothelial NOS (eNOS). Nebivolol produces endothelium-dependent vasodilation by increasing NO release, decreasing oxidative stress to increase NO bioavailability, or both. The NO-dependent vasodilatory action of nebivolol, coupled with its high beta(1)-adrenergic receptor selectivity, is unique among the clinically available beta-blockers and contributes to its efficacy and improved tolerability (e.g., less fatigue and sexual dysfunction) as an antihypertensive agent. (Gupta, Wright, 2008)

Erectile dysfunction

Most cases of erectile dysfunction (ED) are allegedly associated with oxidative stress risk factors such as diabetes mellitus, smoking, hypercholesterolemia and hypertension. **Pomegranate extract significantly improved intracavernosal blood flow, erectile activity, smooth muscle relaxation and fibrosis of the atherosclerotic group in comparison with the atherosclerotic group receiving placebo, but did not normalize them to the age-matched control levels.** (Zhang et al, 2011)

Hypercholesterolemia is an example of antioxidant overkill and it causes erectile dysfunction.

Antioxidant therapy in the treatment of male infertility: an overview

Many studies have focused on the effect of oxidative stress, reactive oxygen species (ROS) and antioxidants on the male productive system. **Under physiological conditions, sperm produces small amounts of EMODs (ROS), which are needed for fertilization, acrosome reaction and capacitation.**

However, if an increased production of EMODs is not associated with a similar increase in scavenging systems, peroxidative damage of the sperm plasma membrane and loss of DNA integrity typically occur, which leads to cell death and reduced fertility.

Furthermore, since there is no linear correlation between sperm quality and pregnancy rates, an improvement in semen parameters should not be the sole outcome considered in studies of antioxidant therapies. **A definitive conclusion regarding the benefit of these therapies is difficult to obtain, as most of the previous studies lacked control groups, considered different antioxidants in different combinations and doses, or did not evaluate pregnancy rates in previously infertile couples.** Even if beneficial effects were reported in a few cases of male infertility, more multi-center, double-blind studies performed with the same criteria are necessary for an increased understanding of the effects of various antioxidants on fertility. Asian Journal of Andrology advance online publication, 20 June 2011; doi:10.1038/aja.2010.183. (Lombardo et al, 2011)

Antioxidants and sperm DNA damage: a clinical perspective

Infertile men possess substantially more sperm DNA damage than do fertile men. Investigators studied and discussed the rationale for antioxidant therapy in men with sperm DNA damage and to evaluate the data on the efficacy of dietary and in vitro antioxidant preparations on sperm DNA damage.

However, the mechanism of action of dietary antioxidants has not been established and most of the clinical studies are small. A beneficial effect of in vitro antioxidant supplements in protecting sperm DNA from exogenous oxidants has been demonstrated, however, **the effect of these antioxidants in protecting sperm from endogenous ROS, gentle sperm processing and cryopreservation has not been established.** (Zini et al, 2009)

Antioxidant therapy in male infertility: fact or fiction?

Infertile men have higher levels of semen reactive oxygen species (ROS, EMODs) than do fertile men. High levels of semen ROS can cause sperm dysfunction, sperm DNA damage and reduced male reproductive potential.

To date, most clinical studies suggest that dietary antioxidant supplements are beneficial in terms of improving sperm function and DNA integrity. However, **the exact mechanism of action of dietary antioxidants and the optimal dietary supplement have not been established.** Moreover, most of the clinical studies are small and few have evaluated pregnancy rates. A beneficial effect of in vitro antioxidant supplements in protecting spermatozoa from exogenous oxidants has been demonstrated in most studies; however, **the effect of these antioxidants in protecting sperm from endogenous ROS, gentle sperm processing and cryopreservation has not been established conclusively.** (Zini, Al-Hathal, 2011)

The role of oxidative stress in spontaneous abortion and recurrent pregnancy loss: a systematic review

Human reproduction is not considered a highly efficient biological process.

It is said that before the end of the first trimester, 30%-50% of conceptions end in spontaneous abortion. Most losses occur at the time of implantation. 15%-20% of clinical pregnancies end in spontaneous abortions.

Recurrent pregnancy loss is a frustrating clinical problem both for clinicians and patients. Recurrent pregnancy loss affects 0.5%-3% of women in the reproductive age group, and between 50%-60% of recurrent pregnancy losses are idiopathic.

The role of antioxidant vitamins for primary prevention of oxidative stress-induced pathologies needs to be investigated further. (Gupta et al, 2007)

CHAPTER SEVENTEEN

Genital infections

Chlamydial infections and EMODs

According to Ramsey et al phagocyte oxidase-derived reactive oxygen species (ROS, EMODs) regulate reactive nitrogen species (RNS) during Chlamydial urogenital infection in the mouse. Ramsey et al further conclude that while neither phagocyte oxidase-derived ROS nor iNOS-derived RNS are essential for resolution of infection, RNS protect from chronic Chlamydial disease in this model. The production of reactive nitrogen species (RNS) through the cytokine-inducible nitric oxide synthase (iNOS) likely plays a contributing role in elimination of Chlamydial infection in vitro, though it is not necessary for resolution of mouse urogenital infection. The IFN-γ-inducible tryptophan decyclizing enzyme 2,3-indoleamine dioxygenase has been shown to restrict Chlamydial growth in human systems in vitro but does not appear to be important in the mouse in response to infection.

In the previous studies, mice deficient in iNOS resolved culture-apparent infection but developed exacerbated disease outcomes as assessed by hydrosalpinx formation and infertility. These observations were concurrent with persistent detection of Chlamydial DNA subsequent to resolution of infection in both $NOS2^{-/-}$ mice and WT mice. While neither phagocyte oxidase-derived ROS nor iNOS-derived RNS are essential for resolution of infection in this model, iNOS-derived RNS protect mice from development of chronic disease as assessed by hydrosalpinx formation.

While the exact mechanisms of disease protection afforded by RNS in this model remain enigmatic, it is rewarding to know that similar roles for free radicals have been reported using different models of inflammatory diseases. The development of several inflammatory diseases of both infectious and noninfectious etiology have been attributed to ROS and RNS individually. The effects of these free radicals on host tissues are multifactoral and include, but are not limited to, enhancement of inflammation through the upregulation of leukocyte adhesion molecules, disruption of normal cellular metabolism, membrane lipid peroxidation, and damage to nucleic acids. When they are considered with the work of Darville et al. that showed an early and prolonged neutrophil influx and associated cytokine production with susceptibility to disease, a plausible hypothesis for our present results could be formed. This would include excessive or protracted inflammatory responses, oxidative tissue damage, and the ensuing chronic disease in the host repair phase in susceptible mice. An increase in RNS production for a resistant strain over that for the susceptible strain could protect from chronic disease development by mollifying the effect of ROS. Indeed, interaction between the two free radical-generating systems seems to provide counter regulatory effects. For example, nitric oxide reacts rapidly with oxygen free radicals to form peroxynitrite and thus modulate the effects of ROS on several cellular systems. Our data showing heightened iNOS activity in the absence of ROS for the $p47^{phox-/-}$ mice support a regulatory role for ROS in controlling the protective activity of iNOS or its product in the murine model. Additionally, ROS and RNS may have opposing and dose-dependent effects on Chlamydia-induced fibrosis through the activation and inhibition of matrix metalloproteinases, which are responsible for extracellular matrix modification and the induction of scarring responses. In general, ROS tend to activate latent matrix metalloproteinases, while RNS may bind the zinc in the their active site, thus inactivating this class of enzymes. Taken together, our results provide support for the hypothesis that the overall balance between superoxide and nitric oxide generation is critical in development of disease subsequent to Chlamydial infection in the mouse model. (Ramsey et al, 2001)

I believe that Ramsey et al are saying that EMODs can be both protective and damaging, in that superoxide can take out nitric oxide by converting it to peroxynitrite.

Male genital tract infections

In the male genital tract, reactive oxygen species (ROS) are generated by spermatozoa and leukocytes including neutrophils and macrophages. **ROS are** involved in the regulation of sperm functions such as capacitation and the acrosome reaction. Infections lead to an excessive ROS production, resulting in an 'oxidative burst' from neutrophils/macrophages as a first-line defense mechanism.

At the site of an infection, the degree of activation of leukocytes, i.e. the amount of ROS produced, and the available antioxidative systems determine whether spermatozoa are damaged or not. During an infection, an imbalance of pro- and antioxidants favoring the former result in oxidative stress which impairs the sperm functions mentioned, as well as motility and fertilization. ROS produced during infections of the testis and epididymis are especially harmful to spermatozoa due to the longer contact time and the lack of antioxidant protection. In the final ejaculate, only very high numbers of ROS-producing leukocytes are detrimental to sperm functions. An infectious injury involving ROS in the prostate gland, seminal vesicles of epididymis could impair sperm functions indirectly. (Ochendorf, 1999)

At this point, Ochendorf is portraying both deliterious and beneficial roles for EMODs.

CHAPTER EIGHTEEN

The role of sperm oxidative stress in male infertility and the significance of oral antioxidant therapy

Oxidative stress in the male germ line is thought to affect male fertility and impact upon normal embryonic development. Accordingly, fertility specialists are actively exploring the diagnosis of such stress in spermatozoa and evaluating the possible use of antioxidants to ameliorate this condition. In this review, evidence for the presence of oxidative stress in human spermatozoa, the origins of this phenomenon, its clinical significance in the etiology of male infertility and recent advances in methods for its diagnosis and treatment are re-examined. Moreover, an extensive review of the results presented in published clinical studies has been conducted to evaluate the overall impact of oral antioxidants on measures of sperm oxidative stress and DNA damage. Administration of antioxidants to infertile men has been assessed in numerous clinical studies with at least 20 reports highlighting its effect on measures of oxidative stress in human spermatozoa. A qualitative but detailed review of the results revealed that **19 of the 20 studies conclusively showed a significant reduction relating to some measure of oxidative stress in these cells. Strong evidence also supports improved motility, particularly in asthenospermic patients. However, of these studies, only 10 reported pregnancy-related outcomes, with 6 reporting positive associations.** Adequately powered, placebo-controlled comprehensive clinical trials are now required to establish a clear role for antioxidants in the prevention of oxidative stress in the male germ line, such that the clinical utility of this form of therapy becomes established once and for all. (Gharagozloo, Aitken, 2011)

Antioxidants and sperm DNA damage: a clinical perspective

Infertile men possess substantially more sperm DNA damage than do fertile men, damage that may impact negatively on reproductive outcomes. In this era of assisted reproductive technologies there is mounting concern regarding the safety of utilizing DNA-damaged spermatozoa in this setting. Therefore, it is important to identify strategies that may reduce sperm DNA damage. The purpose of this review is to discuss the rationale for antioxidant therapy in men with sperm DNA damage and to evaluate the data on the efficacy of dietary and in vitro antioxidant preparations on sperm DNA damage. METHODS: We reviewed the literature on antioxidants and sperm DNA damage. RESULTS: To date, the data suggest that dietary antioxidants may be beneficial in reducing sperm DNA damage, particularly, in men with high levels of DNA fragmentation. However, the mechanism of action of dietary antioxidants has not been established and most of the clinical studies are small. A beneficial effect of in vitro antioxidant supplements in protecting sperm DNA from exogenous oxidants has been demonstrated, however, **the effect of these antioxidants in protecting sperm from endogenous ROS, gentle sperm processing and cryopreservation has not been established.** (Zini et al, 2009)

The etiology of sperm DNA damage is multi-factorial and may be due to primary testicular or secondary (e.g. environmental) factors. **Sperm DNA damage is believed to be the result of aberrant protamine expression, excessive ROS (reactive oxygen species) generation and abortive apoptosis during spermatogenesis.**

The association between sperm DNA damage and semen ROS is the basis for the use of antioxidants in the treatment of sperm DNA damage. **High levels of ROS have been detected in the semen of 25% of infertile men.** (Iwasaki, Gagnon, 1992) (Zini et al, 1993)

The levels of sperm-derived ROS (measured in sperm preparations having minimal leukocyte contamination) have been associated with sperm DNA damage, although **no ROS threshold level above which sperm DNA damage is detected has been established.** (Irvine et al, 2000) (Barroso et al, 2000) (Saleh et al, 2003)

Moreover, **the levels of sperm DNA oxidation are higher in infertile compared to fertile men.** (Shen et al, 1999) (Kodama et al, 1997)

Semen ROS are generated by spermatozoa (especially, defective or immature) and semen leukocytes. (Aitken, Fisher, 1994)

While **the controlled release of low levels of ROS is necessary for normal sperm function**, high levels of ROS can cause sperm dysfunction. (Aitken, Fisher, 1994)

The susceptibility of human spermatozoa to oxidative stress stems primarily from the abundance of unsaturated fatty acids in the sperm plasma membrane. These unsaturated fatty acids provide fluidity that is necessary for membrane fusion events (e.g. the acrosome reaction and sperm-egg interaction) and for sperm motility. However, the unsaturated nature of these molecules predisposes them to free radical attack and ongoing lipid peroxidation throughout the sperm plasma membrane. Once this process has been initiated, accumulation of lipid peroxides occurs on the sperm surface and oxidative damage to DNA can ensue. Studies have demonstrated that exogenous and endogenous ROS can induce sperm DNA damage in vitro, confirming that **ROS may play a role in the etiology of sperm DNA damage in infertile men.** (Twigg et al, 1998) (Aitken et al, 1998) (Sawyer et al, 2003)

Semen antioxidants and sperm DNA damage

Seminal fluid is an important source of antioxidants (ROS scavengers) and is key in protecting spermatozoa from oxidative injury. (Gagnon et al, 1991) (Jeulin et al, 1989)

This is particularly important because **spermatozoa have little cytoplasmic fluid (antioxidant enzymes are generally intracellular), virtually no capacity for protein synthesis and little antioxidant capacity.** (Zini et al, 1993)

RMH Note: How could evolution have gotten it so wrong? If sperm are so sensitive to EMODs, the seminal fluid and sperm should have developed high antioxidant capacities. But they did not!

The endogenous free radical scavenging enzymes in the male reproductive tract include superoxide dismutase (SOD), catalase, and glutathione peroxidase (GPX). (Zini et al, 1993) (Zini et al, 1996) (Jow et al, 1993) (Zini et al, 1997)

These same antioxidant enzymes (SOD, catalase and GPX) are found in semen. (Sanocka et al, 1997)

Moreover, **several non-enzymatic antioxidants (e.g. vitamins C and E, hypotaurine, taurine, L-carnitine, lycopene) are also found in semen** and this non-enzymatic component accounts for much of the total seminal antioxidant activity. (Holmes et al, 1992) (Zini et al, 1993)

Several clinical studies have evaluated the relationship between semen antioxidant levels and sperm DNA damage and have reported conflicting results. Some studies have shown that a deficiency in semen antioxidants is associated with sperm DNA damage, whereas, other studies have not observed such a relationship.

Similarly, **some studies have found that seminal antioxidant activity is reduced in infertile men with high levels of seminal ROS** (relative to those with normal levels of ROS) whereas others have not shown this. (Zini et al, 1993)

To date, there are no studies to indicate a relationship between systemic antioxidant or vitamin deficiency and male infertility. Silver et al, 2005 evaluated a cohort of fertile men and did not identify any relationships between dietary antioxidant intake (vitamins C, E or ß-carotene) and sperm DNA damage.

Nonetheless, it is possible that a subset of infertile men may be at risk for antioxidant deficiency, particularly, vitamin C deficiency. (Hampl et al, 2004)

Moreover, infertile men with specific lifestyles may also be at risk for antioxidant or vitamin deficiency (e.g. smoking, increased alcohol intake, dieting. (Jacob, 1990) (Ryle, Thompson, 1984)

In order to be active, a dietary antioxidant should be effectively absorbed and concentrated in reproductive tract organs. The antioxidant should also replete a deficiency (in the testis, epididymis or semen) and play a role in reproductive function. The antioxidant must either improve spermatogenesis and/or epididymal function, ultimately, resulting in improved sperm function and chromatin compaction and integrity. Alternatively, the antioxidant should enhance semen antioxidant capacity in order to reduce oxidative DNA damage.

There are a small number of reports on the effects of dietary antioxidant supplementation on sperm DNA integrity. In general, these are small studies that do not evaluate the mechanism of action of antioxidants: the only endpoint that is measured is the integrity of the sperm DNA or pregnancy rate. Moreover, most studies evaluate the effects of a short treatment course (with no long-term follow-up), are not randomized and fail to include a placebo-control group. Most of these clinical studies have evaluated men with high levels of sperm DNA damage. In these men, **treatment with antioxidant supplements is generally associated with reduced levels of sperm DNA integrity and/ or improved fertility potential** (Kodama et al, 1997) (Greco, Romano et al, 2005) (Greco, Iacobelli, 2005) (Menezo et al, 2007) (Tremellen et al, 2007) (Gil-Villa et al, 2008) (Piomboni et al, 2008)

In 1991, Fraga et al. demonstrated that dietary vitamin C increases semen vitamin C levels and improves sperm DNA integrity (lowers DNA oxidation levels) in men with a vitamin C deficiency (on a vitamin C depleted diet). More recent studies of infertile men with high levels of sperm DNA damage (**2 randomized controlled and 3 uncontrolled trials) have shown that antioxidant therapy is effective in improving sperm DNA integrity or pregnancy rates.**

In men with unselected infertility, the effect of dietary antioxidants on sperm DNA integrity is equivocal with only one of two controlled trials showing a benefit of antioxidants on sperm DNA integrity.

In vitro antioxidants and sperm DNA damage

Several studies have examined the role of in vitro antioxidant supplementation in protecting the sperm DNA from oxidative damage. This is clinically relevant as sperm washing is routinely performed prior to ARTs (e.g. intrauterine insemination and in vitro fertilization) and the process may result in injury to the sperm DNA, particularly, **as spermatozoa are now vulnerable to oxidative stress because seminal plasma (rich in antioxidants) has been removed in the process.** (Twigg, Irvine, 1998)

However, it is important to note that **subpopulations of spermatozoa will exhibit variable susceptibility to oxidative stress:** the DNA of normal spermatozoa is reportedly less susceptible to gentle processing techniques than is the DNA of abnormal or immature spermatozoa. (Said et al, 2005)

The studies on in vitro antioxidant supplementation have looked at the role of antioxidants in protecting sperm from exogenous and endogenous ROS, and, from the effects of semen processing and cryopreservation. **Antioxidants (e.g. vitamins C and E, catalase, glutathione) have been shown quite clearly to** protect sperm DNA from the effects of exogenous ROS. (Lopes et al, 1998) (Potts et al, 2000) (Sierens et al, 2002) (Russo et al, 2006)

This is of clinical relevance as many of the semen samples contain leukocytes and these cells have the potential to generate exogenous ROS.

In contrast, **antioxidants appear to be of limited value in protecting the DNA of normal spermatozoa from endogenous ROS production (e.g. NADPH-induced or centrifugation-induced)** (Cemeli et al, 2004) (Dobrzynska et al, 2004) (Anderson et al, 2003)

In samples with poor morphology and poor sperm chromatin compaction, antioxidants may protect the sperm DNA from endogenous ROS production, as these samples are more vulnerable to oxidative stress. In general, **antioxidants appear to be of limited value in protecting sperm DNA from gentle semen processing (e.g. incubation or density-gradient centrifugation).** (Chi et al, 2008) (Donnelly et al, 1999) (Hughes et al, 1998) (Donnelly et al, 2000)

In some cases, antioxidants supplementation in vitro (e.g. combination of vitamins C and E) may cause sperm DNA damage. (Donnelly et al, 1999) (Hughes et al, 1998)

The one study evaluating the effects of sperm cryopreservation suggests that antioxidants (vitamin E) do not protect sperm DNA in this setting. (Taylor et al, 2009)

In summary, the data suggest that ROS appear to play an important role in the generation of sperm DNA damage. **Although in vitro studies have demonstrated a beneficial effect of antioxidant supplements in protecting sperm DNA from exogenous oxidants, the effect of these antioxidants in protecting sperm from endogenous ROS, gentle sperm processing and cryopreservation has not been established.** The data suggest that dietary antioxidants may be beneficial in reducing sperm DNA damage, particularly, in men with high levels of DNA fragmentation. However, the mechanism of action of dietary antioxidants has not been established and most of the clinical studies are small. (Zini et al, 2009)

CHAPTER NINETEEN

The origin of human sperm DNA damage

DNA damage in the male germ line has been linked with a variety of adverse clinical outcomes including impaired fertility, an increased incidence of miscarriage and an enhanced risk of disease in the offspring. The origins of this DNA damage could, in principle, involve: (i) abortive apoptosis initiated post meiotically when the ability to drive this process to completion is in decline (ii) unresolved strand breaks created during spermiogenesis to relieve the torsional stresses associated with chromatin remodelling and (iii) **oxidative stress.** They present a two-step hypothesis for the origins of DNA damage in human spermatozoa that highlights the significance of oxidative stress acting on vulnerable, poorly protaminated cells generated as a result of defective spermiogenesis. They further propose that these defective cells are characterized by several hallmarks of 'dysmaturity' including the retention of excess residual cytoplasm, persistent nuclear histones, poor zona binding and disrupted chaperone content. **The oxidative stress experienced by these cells may originate from infiltrating leukocytes or, possibly, the entry of spermatozoa into an apoptosis-like cascade characterized by the mitochondrial generation of reactive oxygen species.** This oxidative stress **may** be exacerbated by a decline in local antioxidant protection, particularly during epididymal maturation. Finally, if oxidative stress is a major cause of sperm DNA damage then **antioxidants should have an important therapeutic role to play** in the clinical management of male infertility. **But this has not been clinically demonstrated or verified. It is still conjecture.** (Aitken, De Luliis, 2010)

Oxidative stress and male infertility

Oxidative stress occurs when the production of potentially destructive reactive oxygen species (ROS) exceeds the bodies own natural antioxidant defenses, resulting in cellular damage. **Oxidative stress is a common pathology seen in approximately half of all infertile men (but what about the other half?).** ROS, defined as including **oxygen ions, free radicals and peroxides are generated by sperm and seminal leukocytes within semen** and produce infertility by two key mechanisms. First, they damage the sperm membrane, decreasing sperm motility and its ability to fuse with the oocyte. Second, ROS can alter the sperm DNA, resulting in the passage of defective paternal DNA on to the conceptus. (Tremellen, 2008)

Mitochondrial functionality in reproduction: from gonads and gametes to embryos and embryonic stem cells

Mitochondria are multitasking organelles involved in ATP synthesis, reactive oxygen species (ROS) production, calcium signalling and apoptosis; and mitochondrial defects are known to cause physiological dysfunction, including infertility. The goal of this review was to identify and discuss common themes in mitochondrial function related to mammalian reproduction.

METHODS The scientific literature was searched for studies reporting on the several aspects of mitochondrial activity in mammalian testis, sperm, oocytes, early embryos and embryonic stem cells.

RESULTS ATP synthesis and ROS production are the most discussed aspects of mitochondrial function. **Metabolic shifts from mitochondria-produced ATP to glycolysis occur at several stages, notably during gametogenesis and early embryo development, either reflecting developmental switches or substrate availability. The exact role of sperm mitochondria is especially controversial.** Mitochondria-generated ROS function in signalling but are mostly described when produced under pathological conditions. Mitochondria-based calcium signalling is primarily important in embryo activation and embryonic stem cell differentiation. Besides pathologically triggered apoptosis, **mitochondria participate in apoptotic events related to the regulation of spermatogonial cell number, as well as gamete, embryo and embryonic stem cell quality.** Interestingly, **data from knock-out (KO) mice is not always straightforward in terms of expected phenotypes.** Finally, recent data suggests that **mitochondrial activity can modulate embryonic stem cell pluripotency as well as differentiation into distinct cellular fates.**

CONCLUSIONS Mitochondria-based events regulate different aspects of reproductive function, but these are not uniform throughout the several systems reviewed. Low mitochondrial activity seems a feature of 'stemness', being described in spermatogonia, early embryo, inner cell mass cells and embryonic stem cells.

(Ramalho-Santos et al, 2009)

Toxicants and human sperm chromatin integrity

The integrity of the paternal genome is essential as the spermatozoon can bring genetic damage into the oocyte at fertilization and contribute to the development of abnormal pregnancy outcome. During the past two decades, many assays have been developed to measure sperm DNA strand breaks, chromatin structure and compaction and assess the proteins associated with the DNA, as well as epigenetic modifications. Using these assays, **it has been shown that exposure to physical agents or chemicals, including therapeutic drugs and environmental toxicants, can affect the integrity of sperm chromatin, inducing structural, genetic and/ or epigenetic abnormalities. The mechanisms by which such damage is triggered are still largely unresolved and the susceptibility of each individual will depend on their genetic background, lifestyle and exposure to various insults. Depending on the nature of the chemicals, they may directly target the DNA, induce an oxidative stress, or modify the epigenetic elements.** The significance of measuring the sperm chromatin integrity comes from the fact that this end-point correlates well with the low IVF and ICSI outcomes, and idiopathic infertility. Nevertheless, **it is hard to establish a direct link between the paternal sperm chromatin integrity and the health of the future generations.** Thus, it seems essential to undertake studies that will resolve the impact of chemical and environmental factors on chromatin structure and epigenetic components of human spermatozoa and to elucidate what sperm nuclear end-points are predictors of the quality of progeny outcome. (Delbes et al, 2010)

Discussion: The role of sperm oxidative stress in male infertility and the significance of oral antioxidant therapy

Oxidative stress in the male germ line is thought to affect male fertility and impact upon normal embryonic development. Accordingly, fertility specialists are actively exploring the diagnosis of such stress in spermatozoa and evaluating the possible use of antioxidants to ameliorate this condition. In this review, evidence for the presence of oxidative stress in human spermatozoa, the origins of this phenomenon, its clinical significance in the aetiology of male infertility and recent advances in methods for its diagnosis and treatment are re-examined. Moreover, an extensive review of the results presented in published clinical studies has been conducted to evaluate the overall impact of oral antioxidants on measures of sperm oxidative stress and DNA damage. Administration of antioxidants to infertile men has been assessed in numerous clinical studies with at least 20 reports highlighting its effect on measures of oxidative stress in human spermatozoa. A qualitative but detailed review of the results revealed that **19 of the 20 studies conclusively showed a significant reduction relating to some measure of oxidative stress in these cells. Strong evidence also supports improved motility, particularly in asthenospermic patients.** However, of these studies, **only 10 reported pregnancy-related outcomes, with 6 reporting positive associations.** Adequately powered, placebo-controlled comprehensive clinical trials are now required to establish a clear role for antioxidants in the prevention of oxidative stress in the male germ line, such that the clinical utility of this form of therapy becomes established once and for all. (Gharagozloo, Aitken, 2011)

Once again, we find inconsistent and confusing results, in that 19 of the 20 clinical studies showed reduction in oxidative stress, only 6 studies reported positive associations with antioxidant therapy and pregnancy related outcomes. Also, **once again, reproducibility of results is lacking** and fails to meet the criteria of the scientific method.

Prevention of oxidative stress injury to sperm

The following discussion was excerpted and modified from: (Agarwal et al, 2005)

The **greatest paradox** of aerobic respiration is that oxygen, which is essential for energy production, may also be detrimental because it leads to the production of reactive oxygen species (ROS, EMODs). When levels of EMODs overwhelm the body's antioxidant defense system, so-called oxidative stress (OS) allegedly occurs. OS is defined as a condition in which the elevated levels of EMODs damage cells, tissues, or organs.

EMODs are free radicals that play a significant role in many of the sperm physiological processes such as capacitation, hyperactivation, and sperm-oocyte fusion. (Aitken et al, 2004) (Allamaneni et al, 2004) (de Lamirande et al, 1998)

However, EMODs also trigger many pathological processes in the male reproductive system, and these processes have been implicated in cancers of the bladder and prostate, as well as in male infertility. (Bankson et al, 1993) (Hietanen et al, 1994) (Agarwal, Saleh, 2002)

Spermatozoa are sensitive to OS because they lack cytoplasmic defenses. (Agarwal, Saleh, 2002)

Moreover, the sperm plasma membrane contains lipids in the form of polyunsaturated fatty acids, which are vulnerable to attack by EMODs. EMODs, in the presence of polyunsaturated fatty acids, were believed to trigger a chain of chemical reactions called lipid peroxidation. However, I believe that this has not occurred in brain tissue and likely does not occur in the testicles.

EMODs can also damage DNA by causing deletions, mutations, and other lethal genetic effects. It is difficult to block the OS-induced injury to cells or tissues because EMODs are continuously produced by cellular aerobic metabolism. (Davies, 2000)

Several clinical trials are currently attempting to minimize the toxic effects of OS on human spermatozoa. (Agarwal, Said, 2004)

Sources of EMODs in Semen

There are two main sources of EMODs in semen: leukocytes and immature spermatozoa. (Garrido et al, 2004)

Of these, leukocytes are considered to be the primary source of EMODs. (Aitken et al, 1992)

Leukocytes, particularly neutrophils and macrophages, have been associated with excessive EMOD production that ultimately leads to sperm dysfunction.

Spermatozoa produce EMODs mainly when a defect occurs during spermio-genesis that results in retention of cytoplasmic droplets. (Gomez et al, 1996) (Zini et al, 1993)

A strong positive correlation exists between immature spermatozoa and EMOD production, which in turn negatively affects the sperm quality.

The two main sites of EMOD production are **the mitochondrion and the sperm plasma membrane.** The mitochondrion is the powerhouse of respiration. Hence, it is the major site of EMOD generation, which is produced through the nicotinamide adenine dinucleotide-dependent oxido-reductase pathway. In contrast, the sperm plasma membrane produces EMODs through the nicotinamide adenine dinucleotide phosphate-dependent oxidase system. Xanthine oxidase—a key enzyme in purine catabolism—is also involved in the production of EMODs in spermatozoa.

Oxidative Damage to Spermatozoa by Life-Style Behaviors

Damage Caused by Pollution— Environmental pollution and radiation can generate various ROS such as hydrogen peroxide (H_2O_2), superoxide anion, and hydroxyl radical. According to an **Italian study on tollgate workers,** traffic pollution damages sperm and may reduce fertility in young and middle-aged men. **The workers in that study showed poorer sperm quality than age-matched men living in the same area who were not exposed to the same level of automobile pollution. In addition, sperm function tests revealed that the workers had less active spermatozoa.** In the subset of workers with abnormal sperm parameters, sperm count and viability were inversely correlated with lead (Pb) levels, whereas sperm motility, viability, membrane function, nuclear DNA integrity, linearity, and amplitude of sperm lateral movement were inversely correlated with methemoglobin levels—a marker for nitrogen oxide.

Damage Caused by Smoking— Smoking induces OS either by increasing levels of oxidants originating from the smoke or by decreasing levels of antioxidants in the seminal plasma. Therefore, **smokers may need to increase their intake of antioxidants to compensate for this deficiency.** According to a study conducted by our group, smoking greatly increases levels of leukocyte and EMODs. Other studies have reported that tobacco adversely affects sperm quality (i.e., concentration, motility, and morphology. Smoking also predominately affects sperm DNA, as evidenced from the increased level of 8-deoxygunosine (8-oxodG)—

a marker for oxidative DNA damage. Therefore, smoking may not affect the fertilization rate per se, but it will increase the risk of heritable mutations.

Oxidative Damage to Spermatozoa by Infection

Sperm damage can be caused either by the invading pathogens or by the defense mechanisms that are employed against them. (Ochsendorf, 1999)

For example, when microorganisms invade the human body, it produces polymorphonuclear leukocytes and macrophages, which are the major sources of ROS production. Prostatitis and accessory gland infection increase OS, which severely damages spermatozoa. In addition, a past infection by the sexually transmitted *Neisseria gonorrhea* is associated with leukocytospermia. Although there is no direct evidence that *Neisseria gonorrhea* directly increases EMOD production, the associated leukocytospermia is well known to produce EMODs.

According to a study by Depuydt et al, leukocytospermia and male accessory glands infection reduce a man's fertilizing potential by affecting sperm parameters both in vitro and in vivo. (Depuydt et al, 1998)

Iatrogenic Oxidative Damage to Spermatozoa

Prolonged in vitro incubation of semen samples that contain high levels of immature spermatozoa before sperm processing increases the risk of OS damage to mature spermatozoa. In a study by Aitken and Clarkson, it was reported that **repeated centrifugation mechanically injures spermatozoa and increases EMOD production. (Aitken, Clarkson, 1988)**

OS may also **damage sperm during cryopreservation**. A study by Bilodeau et al revealed that EMODs generated during freeze-thaw cycles are detrimental to sperm function and that levels of antioxidants were diminished during each cycle. (Bilodeau et al, 2000)

I believe that this opens up these studies to considerable artifacts during the studies themselves and values obtained may not represent actual EMODs produced by sperm.

Strategies for OS Prevention

Antioxidants— **Antioxidants are the main defense against OS induced by free radicals.** There are prevention antioxidants and scavenger antioxidants. Prevention antioxidants such as metal chelators and metal-binding proteins block the formation of new EMODs, whereas scavenger antioxidants remove the EMODs that have already formed.

Prevention Antioxidants— Transition metal ions, mainly iron, are involved in the generation of the highly reactive ˙OH by Fenton's reaction. They stimulate lipid peroxidation by decomposing the peroxides into peroxyl and alkoxyl radicals, which in turn causes the chain reaction of lipid peroxidation. **Metal chelators such as transferrin, lactoferrin, and ceruloplasmin** that are present in human semen control lipid peroxidation of the sperm plasma membrane, protecting its integrity.

Other metal chelators such as ethylene diamine tetraacetic acid, 1,10-phen-anthrolin, and neocuproine have been shown to reduce sperm DNA damage in fishes. However, **similar data are lacking in human.**

In vitro supplementation of **metal chelators such as DL-penicillamine, 2,3-dimercaptopropan-I sulphonate and meso-2,3-dimercapto-succinimic acid** showed enhancement of sperm quality during assisted reproductive technique. In a study by Wroblewski et al, incubating sperm with D-penicillamine significantly increased sperm motility.

Cadmium (Cd), a class B element, is capable of replacing zinc, thereby exerting its toxic effect in spermatogenesis. **Metallothionein removes Cd from the body** by binding to it, which results in improved spermatogenesis, maturation, and capacitation of spermatozoa.

Scavenger Antioxidants— **Dietary antioxidants form an essential part of the human antioxidant defense system.** Fruits and vegetables as well as daily dietary supplements constitute the potential sources of various antioxidants. The National Academy of Sciences has recommended 60 mg vitamin C per day for an adult male. The daily requirement of vitamin E varies from 50 to 800 mg, depending on the intake of fruits, vegetables, tea, or wine. Carotenoids and selenium work synergistically with vitamin E and have a recommended dietary allowances value of 1000 and 70 micrograms per day, respectively. (National Academy of

Sciences. *Recommended Dietary Allowances.* 10th ed. National Academy Press. 1989). I believe that these numbers are outdated and rather meaningless.

Oxidative stress may also be limited by using chain-breaking antioxidants such as vitamin E and vitamin C as drug supplements. **Vitamin C is a major chain-breaking antioxidant and is present in the extracellular fluid. It neutralizes hydroxyl, superoxide, and hydrogen peroxide radicals and prevents sperm agglutination. In addition, it also helps recycle vitamin E.**

Vitamin C is found in reduced quantity in the seminal plasma of infertile men. (Lewis et al, 1997)

Vitamin C increases sperm counts in vivo in infertile male patients with oral doses ranging from 200-1000 mg/day. (Dawson et al, 1987)

The combination of flavonoids and vitamin C increases the effectiveness of both of these compounds. They conserve the alpha-tocopherol content of low-density lipoprotein and delay the onset of lipid peroxidation. **Quercetin and xanthohumol** constitute some of the important dietary flavonoids.

The principal chain-breaking antioxidant vitamin E is present within the cell membrane. It neutralizes H_2O_2 and protects the plasma membrane from lipid peroxidation. In a randomized cross-over study, oral administration of 600 mg/day of vitamin E improved sperm function as assessed by the zona binding test. (Kessopoulou et al, 1995)

Selenium is a necessary component for the synthesis of glutathione peroxidase. It works synergistically with vitamin E. According to a study conducted by Keskes-Ammar et al, 225 µg/day of selenium and 400 mg/day of vitamin E oral supplementation for 3 months significantly decreased malondialdehyde concentrations in seminal plasma and improved sperm motility. (Keskes-Ammar et al, 2003)

However **these findings were not confirmed in another study. Selenium supplementation enhances the element concentration in blood and seminal fluid but does not change the spermatozoal quality characteristics in sub-fertile men.** (Iwanier, Zachara, 1995). **Here we go with the inconsistencies again.**

Carotenoids such as beta-carotene and lycopene also form an important component of the antioxidant defense. Beta-carotenes protect the plasma membrane against lipid peroxidation. Lycopene is found in abundance in tomatoes and has a suggested daily intake of 5-10 mg/day. Lycopene has been shown to be twice as potent as beta-carotene and 10 times more potent than vitamin E in scavenging singlet oxygen and inhibiting lipid peroxidation in serum plasma. (Di Mascio et al, 1989)

Glutathione is the most abundant antioxidant found in the body. It plays an important role in protecting lipids, proteins, and nucleic acids against oxidative damage. It combines with vitamin E and selenium to form glutathione peroxidase. In a placebo-controlled, double-blind, cross-over trial, 600 mg glutathione was administered for 2 months by intramuscular injection in 20 infertile men. Glutathione therapy significantly increased sperm motility, particularly forward progression. (Lenzi et al, 1993)

Coenzyme Q-10 (CoQ-10) found in the sperm mid-piece recycles vitamin E, prevents its prooxidant activity, and is also involved in energy production. In a study conducted on 32 infertile males, CoQ-10 inhibited H_2O_2 formation in seminal fluid and in seminal plasma. (Alleva et al, 1997)

In an in vitro study on 22 semen samples of asthenozoospermic men, incubation with 50 μM of CoQ-10 significantly increased sperm motility. In the same study, in vivo supplementation of 60 mg of CoQ-10 in 17 infertile men improved their fertilization rate without changing their semen parameters. (Lewin, Lavon, 1997)

Zinc and copper are trace metals that constitute a part of superoxide dismutase—a key enzymatic antioxidant. Their adequate intake is necessary to maintain the optimal functioning level of these enzymes. At present, it is estimated that the average daily intake in United States is 12.3 mg of zinc and 900 μg of copper per person. Caution should be exercised during intake of these trace metals because some of them can catalyze the reactions that lead to the formation of ROS. An in vitro study by Lloyd et al on salmon sperm DNA determined that at concentrations of 20-50 μM and above, these metal ions caused a maximum DNA strand breaks. No such studies are available in humans, and the in vivo dosage required for these concentrations in seminal plasma is still unknown.

Other antioxidants may also protect against OS, such as **alpha lipoic acid and carnitines.** Alpha lipoic acid (thiols) undergoes reduction to form dihydrolipoic acid, thereby regenerating other antioxidants such as vitamins C and E and reduced glutathione through redox cycling. In contrast, **carnitines are dietary antioxidants that decrease ROS by removing excess intracellular toxic acetyl-CoA that are responsible for mitochondrial ROS production.** Carnitines also improve sperm motility.

However, the positive effects of antioxidants are still debatable. **Multiple studies have found no improvement following antioxidant intake.** (Agarwal et al, 2004) (Ford, Whittington, 1998) (Martin-Du Pan, Sakkas, 1998) (Moilanen, Hovatta, 1995) (Rolf et al, 1999)

Another study (Rolf et al, 1999) **failed to show a positive effect of antioxidants improving ejaculate parameters (volume, concentration, motility, viability),** however this study did not address fertilization or pregnancy rates.

Prevention of Iatrogenic Oxidative Damage— The use of specific sperm preparation techniques has greatly reduced the OS associated with sperm handling and cryopreservation. Sperm separation techniques such as migration-sedimentation, density centrifugation gradient, and glass-wool filtration significantly reduce the level of EMODs by removing leukocytes, which are the major source of EMODs.

In vitro supplements used during sperm preparation and assisted reproductive technique also help to protect spermatozoa against EMODs. Moreover, adding antioxidants to the culture media neutralizes EMODs produced by the leukocytes and immature spermatozoa and improves spermoocyte fusion.

In an in vitro study, **rebamipide effectively scavenged EMODs** during sperm processing and cryopreservation. In another study performed on samples from 25 male partners of infertile couples, in vitro supplementation with superoxide dismutase and catalase prevented lipid peroxidation of the sperm plasma membrane by EMODs and contributed to the recovery of high-quality spermatozoa after freezing-thawing procedures. Similarly, it has been found that **adding glutathione and hypotaurine protects spermatozoa against oxidative damage induced by H_2O_2.** (Donnelly et al, 2000)

Pentoxifylline—a methylxanthine derivative that inhibits phosphodiesterase—has been approved by the US Food and Drug Administration for use in humans. It has a beneficial effect on sperm motility and acrosome reaction and reduces the superoxide release by the human spermatozoa.

N-acetyl-L-cysteine—a precursor of glutathione—reduces the EMOD production in human ejaculate, as well as EMOD-induced DNA damage. The use of vitamin E in vitro has been also documented to improve sperm motility and viability. Hughes et al have determined that in vitro supplementation of vitamins C, E, and urate separately has protective effects on sperm DNA integrity on irradiation. (Hughes et al, 1998)

I guess that they are trying to tell me that any condition which has high antioxidant levels, such as hypercholesterolemia, hyperuricemia, hyperbilirubinemia and excess levels of estrogens and testosterone, will also improve sperm function and integrity. I do not believe it.

Conclusions

Spermatozoa are under a continuous influence of OS because of excessive generation of EMODs.

Although spermatozoa are affected in different ways by OS, there are sufficient antioxidant protections that can decrease the progression of the damage. However, when an imbalance exists between levels of EMODs and the natural antioxidant defenses, various measures can be used to protect spermatozoa against the OS-induced injury. Diet forms an important component of the antioxidant protection system; it supplies the major antioxidants such vitamin C, vitamin E, and carotenoids. Therefore, food rich in these elements should form a part of the daily diet. For those patients who are suspected to have high levels of EMODs, **antioxidant supplements can be considered.** Nevertheless, **further studies are required to validate their use in this group of patients.** In certain cases, it is also essential to modify certain lifestyle behaviors because many habits and environmental factors increase the production of EMODs and affect fertility.

Another important method for decreasing OS is the use of antioxidants during various sperm processing techniques. Antioxidants decrease the oxidative damage to spermatozoa induced during these techniques. There **are many controversies** regarding the doses, types, and combinations that could be used in different sperm-handling techniques.

Male reproductive senescence: the price of immune-induced oxidative damage on sexual attractiveness in the blue-footed booby

In animals, male reproduction is commonly a function of sexual attractiveness, based on the expression of sexually dimorphic traits that advertise genuinely the male's quality. Male performance may decline with age because physiological functions underlying sexual attractiveness may be affected by senescence. Here **we show that a sexual signal (foot color) declines with age, due probably to the deleterious effects of oxidative damage.** We found that in the blue-footed booby Sula nebouxii foot color during courtship was less attractive in senescent than in middle-aged males. In addition, we increased reactive oxygen species experimentally by immunizing males with lipopolysaccharide, a bacterial cell wall component that induces marked oxidative stress in animals. **The immune system activation induced greater lipid peroxidation and invoked changes on color expression (less attractive), particularly in senescent males.** These results support the idea that **oxidative stress affects reproductive senescence,** and suggest that **oxidative damage might be a proximal mechanism underlying age-reproductive patterns in long-lived animals.** (Torres, Velando 2007)

A multifaceted approach to maximize erectile function and vascular health

Daily moderate exercise stimulates vascular NO production. Maintenance of normal body weight and waist/hip ratio allows NO stimulation by insulin. Decreased intake of fat, sugar, and simple carbohydrates rapidly converted to sugar reduces the adverse effects of fatty acids and sugar on endothelial NO production. Omega-3 fatty acids stimulate endothelial NO release. Antioxidants boost NO production and prevent NO breakdown. Folic acid, calcium, vitamin C, and vitamin E support the biochemical pathways leading to NO release. Cessation of smoking and avoidance of excessive alcohol preserve normal endothelial function. **Moderate use of alcohol and certain proprietary supplements may favorably influence erectile and vascular function. Treatment of any remaining testosterone deficit will both increase erectile function and reduce any associated metabolic syndrome.** After production of NO and cyclic GMP are improved, use of **phosphodiesterase-5 inhibitors should result in greater success in treating remaining erectile dysfunction.** Recent studies have also suggested positive effects of phosphodiesterase-5 inhibitors on vascular function. CONCLUSION(S): A multifaceted approach will maximize both erectile function and vascular health. (Meldrum et al, 2010)

Nitric oxide and penile erectile function

The discovery of nitric oxide (NO) as an intercellular messenger or neurotransmitter opened a new era for identifying the important mechanisms underlying physiological and pathophysiological events in autonomically innervated organs and tissues; it also provided the way for development of new therapeutics based on a novel concept of molecule and cell interaction. Endothelium-derived relaxing factor (EDRF) discovered by Furchgott and Zawadzki has been proved to be NO, a labile gaseous molecule, that modulates vascular tone, platelet aggregation and adhesion, and vascular smooth muscle proliferation. Later, NO was determined to act as a non-adrenergic, non-cholinergic (NANC) neurotransmitter of postganglionic parasympathetic nerve fibers, innervating a variety of smooth muscles including the penile corpus cavernosum (CC). The nerve is called "nitrergic" or "nitroxidergic". Although CC sinusoidal endothelial cells also produce and liberate NO in response to chemical and possibly physical stimuli, roles of neurogenic NO in penile erection appear to be more attractive and convincing. NO is formed from L-arginine via catalysis by NO synthase (NOS) isoforms, neuronal (nNOS), endothelial (eNOS), and inducible NOS. NO from nerves and possibly endothelia plays a crucial role in initiating and maintaining intracavernous pressure increase, penile vasodilatation, and penile erection that are dependent on cyclic GMP synthesized with activation of soluble guanylyl cyclase by NO in smooth muscle cells. Erectile dysfunction (ED) is caused by a variety of pathogenic factors, particularly impaired formation and action of NO. Thus, replenishment of this molecule or intracellular cyclic GMP is expected so far to be the most promising therapeutic measures for patients with ED. This article includes recent advances in research on physiological roles and pathophysiological implications of NO in penile erection and on novel therapy for ED in reference to NO. (Toda et al, 2005)

I believe that excessive antioxidant levels establish a symbiotic host-cancer redox micro-environment. Thus, XS AOX is the carcinogenesis etiopathogenesis due to a resultant pro-tumorous EMOD insufficiency state.

NO produced within mitochondria under normal conditions may serve a regulatory purpose, but when generated in excess, such as during inflammation, it may inhibit respiration and ATP production. According to Leon et al. and Maldonado et al., melatonin has been shown to inhibit NOS. .

RMH: Thus, I ask, "What effect could this (inhibition of NOS synthesis) have on male penile erections?" (Reiter et al, 2008)

Study Finds Antioxidants Boost Male Fertility

Researchers at The University of Western Australia and Monash University have discovered **dietary antioxidants can help maintain male fertility.**

Dr Maria Almbro and Winthrop Professor Leigh Simmons, from UWA's Centre for Evolutionary Biology, and Dr Damian Dowling, from Monash University's School of Biological Sciences, studied **crickets and found that a combination of antioxidants provided the best weapon to boost the health of the male ejaculate.** The study was published today in the prestigious journal *Ecology Letters*.

Professor Simmons said highly reactive molecules, known as **free radicals were waste products of the cellular processes that fuel the body's activities.** "These free radicals damage cells if they are not neutralized by antioxidants," he said.

Dr Almbro said sperm were known to be vulnerable to attack from free radicals, and the study had shown that **the best defense against sperm damage was to take two antioxidants; Vitamin E and beta-carotene.**

Professor Simmons said for most animals, it was typical for females to have the sperm of several males inside them at any given time, competing for the fertilization of the eggs.

"It is fair to say that the sperm are at war within the female, and we can expect that the most competitive sperm will win the race to the egg. Our study showed that the **sperm of males who were fed antioxidants were easily able to outclass the sperm of rival males who were deprived of antioxidants.**"

Dr Dowling said medical scientists had already provided evidence that antioxidants were important in maintaining sperm health.

"What we have done is provide a definitive experimental confirmation of this, not in a test tube, but in a real living animal, showing that **antioxidants are profoundly important in deciding the outcomes of reproduction in males.**

"That is to say, **antioxidants in the diet equal more babies, at least in these crickets.** And by working with crickets rather than humans as subjects, we were able to conduct the experiment under very strictly controlled conditions - ruling out all other alternative explanations for our results."

The researchers will now determine the precise mechanism by which dietary antioxidants enhance male fertility in these insects.

http://insciences.org/article.php?article_id=10230. Accessed 8-8-11.

CHAPTER TWENTY

Sperm may be harmed by exposure to the antioxidant, BPA, study suggests

ANN ARBOR, Mich.—In one of the first human studies of its kind, researchers have found that urinary concentrations of the controversial chemical **Bisphenol A, or BPA, may be related to decreased sperm quality and sperm concentration.**

However, the researchers are quick to point out that these results are preliminary and more study is needed. Several studies have documented adverse effects of BPA on semen in rodents, but none are known to have reported similar relationships in humans.

BPA is a common chemical that's stirred much controversy in the media lately over its safety. Critics say that BPA mimics the body's own hormones and may lead to negative health effects. **BPA is most commonly used to make plastics and epoxy resins used in food and beverage cans, and people are exposed primarily through diet, although other routes are possible.**

More than 6 billion pounds of BPA are produced annually.

BPA is an antioxidant

The new study suggests that more research should focus on BPA and health effects in adults, says John Meeker, assistant professor of Environmental Health Sciences at the University of Michigan School of Public Health.

Meeker is the lead author on the study, along with Russ Hauser, the Frank Lee Hisaw Professor of Reproductive Physiology at Harvard School of Public

Health. Colleagues at Massachusetts General Hospital and the U.S. Centers for Disease Control and Prevention also contributed to the research.

"Much of the focus for BPA is on the exposures in utero or in early life, which is of course extremely important, but this suggests exposure may also be a concern for adults," Meeker said. "Research should focus on impacts of exposure throughout multiple life stages."

Meeker and Hauser recruited **190 men** through a fertility clinic. All gave spot urine samples and sperm samples the same day. Subsequently, 78 of the men gave one or two additional urine samples a month apart. **Researchers detected BPA in 89 percent of the urine samples.**

Researchers measured sperm concentration, sperm motility, sperm shape and DNA damage in the sperm cell.

"We found that if we compare somebody in the top quartile of exposure with the lowest quartile of exposure, **sperm concentration was on average about 23 percent lower in men with the highest BPA**," Meeker said.

Results also suggested a 10 percent increase in sperm DNA damage.

The results are consistent with a previous study by Meeker and Hauser suggesting that certain hormones, specifically **FSH (follicle-stimulating hormone) and Inhibin B, are elevated or decreased in relation to BPA**, respectively, **a pattern consistent with low sperm production and development.**

Meeker stressed that further study is necessary due to the study's relatively small sample size and design.

"The study from which these data came is currently in progress," Hauser said. "With a larger sample size and enhanced study design, we will be able to more definitively investigate this preliminary association in the near future."

The Paper: Semen quality and sperm DNA damage in relation to urinary bisphenol A among men from an infertility clinic

http://insciences.org/article.php?article_id=9372. accessed 8-8-11.

Semen quality and sperm DNA damage in relation to urinary bisphenol A among men from an infertility clinic (Meeker et al, 2010) (#190)

Bisphenol A (BPA) (an antioxidant) impairs spermatogenesis in animals, but human studies are lacking. We measured urinary BPA concentrations, semen quality, and sperm DNA damage (comet assay) in 190 men recruited through an infertility clinic. BPA was detected in 89% of samples, with a median (interquartile range [IQR]) concentration of 1.3 (0.8-2.5) ng/mL. Urinary BPA concentration was associated with slightly elevated, though not statistically significant, odds for below reference sperm concentration, motility, and morphology. When modeled as continuous dependent variables, an IQR increase in urinary BPA concentration was associated with declines in sperm concentration, motility, and morphology of 23% (95%CI -40%, -0.3%), 7.5% (-17%, +1.5%), and 13% (-26%, -0.1%), respectively, along with a 10% (0.03%, 19%) increase in sperm DNA damage measured as the percentage of DNA in comet tail. In conclusion, *urinary BPA may be associated with declined semen quality and increased sperm DNA damage*, but confirmatory studies are needed. (Meeker et al, 2010)

Reactive oxygen species and boar sperm function

Boar spermatozoa are very susceptible to reactive oxygen species (ROS), **but ROS involvement in damage and/or capacitation is unclear.** The impact of exposing fresh boar spermatozoa to an ROS-generating system (xanthine/ xanthine oxidase; XA/XO) on sperm ROS content, membrane lipid peroxidation, phospholipase (PL) A activity, and motility, viability, and capacitation was contrasted to ROS content and sperm function after cryopreservation. Exposing boar sperm (n = 4-5 ejaculates) to the ROS-generating system for 30 min rapidly increased hydrogen peroxide ($H2O2$) and lipid peroxidation in all sperm, increased PLA in dead sperm, and did not affect intracellular $O2-$ (flow cytometry of sperm labeled with 2',7'-dichlorodihydrofluorscein diacetate, BODIPY 581/591 CII, bis-BODIPY-FL CII, hydroethidine, respectively; counterstained for viability). Sperm viability remained high, but sperm became immotile. **Cryopreservation decreased sperm motility, viability, and intracellular $O2-$ significantly, but did not affect $H2O2$.** As expected, more sperm incubated in capacitating media than Beltsville thawing solution buffer underwent acrosome reactions and protein tyrosine phosphorylation (four proteins, 58-174 kDa); which proteins were tyrosine phosphorylated was pH dependent. Pre-exposing sperm to the ROS-generating system increased the percentage of sperm that underwent acrosome reactions after incubation in capacitating conditions (P < 0.025), and decreased capacitation-dependent increases in two tyrosine-phosphorylated proteins (P < or = 0.035). In summary, **$H2O2$ is the** major free radical mediating direct ROS effects, but not cryopreservation changes, on boar sperm. Boar sperm motility, acrosome integrity, and lipid peroxidation are more sensitive indicators of oxidative stress than viability and PLA activity. ROS may stimulate the acrosome reaction in boar sperm through membrane lipid peroxidation and PLA activation. (Awda et al, 2009)

Semen analysis and sperm function assays: what do they mean?

Appropriate laboratory testing is an integral component of the proper evaluation of the male presenting with infertility. This article reviews the semen analysis and sperm function assays. Sperm function testing is used to determine if the sperm have the biologic capacity to perform the tasks necessary to reach and fertilize ova and ultimately result in live births. **For a sperm to be fertile in vivo, it must be able to traverse the cervical mucus and reach the ova. The sperm must undergo capacitation and the acrosome reaction, fuse with the oolemma, and incorporate into the ooplasm.** Proper embryo development requires that functional DNA be delivered to the ooplasm. Defects in any of these steps may result in infertility. A variety of tests are available to evaluate different aspects of these functions. To accurately use these functional assays, the clinician must understand what the tests measure, what the indications are for the assays, and how to interpret the results to direct further testing or patient management. (Sigman et al, 2009)

CHAPTER TWENTY ONE

The following paper by Zini was used as a frame work for this section of my book. (Zini et al, 2009)

Antioxidants and sperm DMA damage: a clinical perspective

Infertile men possess substantially more sperm DNA damage than do fertile men, damage that may impact negatively on reproductive outcomes. In this era of assisted reproductive technologies there is mounting concern regarding the safety of utilizing DNA-damaged spermatozoa in this setting. Therefore, it is important to identify strategies that may reduce sperm DNA damage. The purpose of this review is to discuss the rationale for antioxidant therapy in men with sperm DNA damage and to evaluate the data on the efficacy of dietary and in vitro antioxidant preparations on sperm DNA damage. METH-ODS: **We reviewed the literature on antioxidants and sperm DNA damage.** RESULTS: To date, the **data suggest that dietary antioxidants** *may be* **beneficial in reducing sperm DNA damage**, particularly, in men with high levels of DNA fragmentation. **However, the mechanism of action of dietary antioxidants has not been established and most of the clinical studies are small. A beneficial effect of in vitro antioxidant supplements in protecting sperm DNA from exogenous oxidants has been demonstrated, however, the effect of these antioxidants in protecting sperm from endogenous EMODs, gentle sperm processing and cryopreservation has not been established.** (Zini et al, 2009)

Let this sink in, "**The effect of these antioxidants in protecting sperm from endogenous EMODs, gentle sperm processing and cryopreservation has not been established.**"

It is believed to be important to identify strategies that may reduce sperm DNA damage. **The proposed strategies include eliminating testicular gonadotoxins or hyperthermia, treatment of semen or genital tract infections, correction of varicoceles and the use of antioxidants.** (Fraga et al, 1991) (Zini et al, 2005) (Ochsendorf, 1999)

I am suspect of the work of Ames in the early 1990s. At that time and shortly thereafter, he was suggesting that EMODs were causative of a host of diseases and aging. These notions have not been supported by current data with any respectable degree of reliability.

Etiology of sperm damage

The etiology of sperm DNA damage is multi-factorial and may be due to primary testicular or secondary (e.g. environmental) factors. Sperm DNA damage is believed to be the result of aberrant protamine expression, **excessive EMOD (reactive oxygen species, EMODs) generation and abortive apoptosis during spermatogenesis.** (Sakkas et al, 2003) (Aitken et al, 2009) (Carrell, Liu, 2001) (de Yebra et al, 1993)

Relationship between EMODs and sperm DNA damage

The association between sperm DNA damage and semen EMODs is the basis for the use of antioxidants in the treatment of sperm DNA damage. High levels of EMODs have been detected in the semen of 25% of infertile men. (Iwasaki, Gagnon, 1992) (Zini et al, 1993)

But, please remember that this may be purely an association and not evidence of causation.

The levels of sperm-derived EMODs (measured in sperm preparations having minimal leukocyte contamination) have been associated with sperm DNA damage, although no EMOD threshold level above which sperm DNA damage is detected has been established. (Irvine et al, 2000) (Barroso et al, 2000) (Saleh et al, 2003)

The latter part of this sentence is of most importance: **"No EMOD threshold level above which sperm DNA damage is detected has been established."**

Moreover, **the levels of sperm DNA oxidation are higher in infertile compared to fertile men.** (Shen et al, 1999) (Kodama et al, 1997)

Again, this may be a spurious association.

Semen EMODs are generated by spermatozoa (especially, defective or immature) and semen leukocytes. (Barroso et al, 2000) (Sati et al, 2008) (Muratori et al, 2000) (Gomez et al, 1996) (Aitken, Fisher, 1994)

While **the controlled release of low levels of EMODs is necessary for normal sperm function,** high levels of ROS can cause sperm dysfunction. (Aitken, Fisher, 1994)

This is also a most important observation, in that "EMODs are necessary for sperm function."

The susceptibility of human spermatozoa to oxidative stress stems primarily (theoretically) from the abundance of unsaturated fatty acids in the sperm plasma membrane. These unsaturated fatty acids provide fluidity that is necessary for membrane fusion events (e.g. the acrosome reaction and sperm-egg interaction) and for sperm motility. However, **the unsaturated nature of these molecules predisposes them to free radical attack and ongoing lipid peroxidation** throughout the sperm plasma membrane. Once this process has been initiated, accumulation of lipid peroxides occurs on the sperm surface and oxidative damage to DNA can ensue. (Alverez et al, 1987) (Twigg et al, 1998)

Studies have demonstrated that exogenous and endogenous EMODs can induce sperm DNA damage in vitro, showing that EMODs *may* play a role in the etiology of sperm DNA damage in infertile men. (Twigg et al, 1998) (Aitken, 1998) (Sawyer et al, 2003)

Semen antioxidants and sperm DNA damage

Seminal fluid is an important source of antioxidants (ROS, EMOD scavengers) and is key in protecting spermatozoa from oxidative injury. (Jeulin et al, 1989) (Gagnon et al, 1991)

This is particularly important because **spermatozoa have little cytoplasmic fluid (antioxidant enzymes are generally intracellular),** virtually no capacity for protein synthesis **and little antioxidant capacity.** (Zini et al, 1993)

I believe that this is because EMODs are essential for proper sperm function. By the Darwinian laws of evolution, sperm would have evolved high levels of antioxidant protection, if EMOD protection was of prime importance for reproduction and perpetuation of the species over eons of time.

The endogenous free radical scavenging enzymes in the male reproductive tract include superoxide dismutase (SOD), catalase, and glutathione peroxidase (GPx). (Zini et al, 1993) (Zini et al, 1996) (Zini, Schlegel, 1997) (Jow et al, 1993) (Zini et al, 1997)

Although I will not discuss it at this point, I have shown that SOD and GPx are prooxidant enzymes, not antioxidant enzymes.

These same antioxidant enzymes (SOD, catalase and GPx) are found in semen. (Sanocka et al, 1997)

Moreover, several non-enzymatic antioxidants (e.g. vitamins C and E, hypotaurine, taurine, L-carnitine, lycopene) are also found in semen and this non-enzymatic component accounts for much of the total seminal antioxidant activity. (Holmes et al, 1992)

Several clinical studies have evaluated the relationship between semen antioxidant levels and sperm DNA damage and have reported conflicting results.

Actually, conflicting results are a hallmark, trait and characteristic for all antioxidant studies.

Some studies have shown that a deficiency in semen antioxidants is associated with sperm DNA damage, whereas, other studies have not observed such a relationship. (Song et al, 2008) (Appasamy et al, 2007) (Verit et at, 2006) (Xu et al, 2003)

Appasamy's study investigated the relationship between male reproductive hormones and sperm DNA damage and markers of oxidative stress in men undergoing infertility evaluation for male factor (n = 66) and non-male factor (n = 63) infertility. Semen samples were analyzed for DNA fragmentation index (DFI). Serum samples were analyzed for FSH, inhibin B, anti-Müllerian hormone (AMH), testosterone and total antioxidant capacity (TAC). Serum inhibin B was significantly lower in the male factor group compared with the non-male factor group. Inhibin B showed a positive correlation with sperm concentration and motility, and serum AMH showed a positive correlation with sperm concentration and semen volume. DFI was 3-fold higher in the male factor group and showed a negative correlation with sperm motility. Blood plasma TAC was negatively related to sperm concentration. The results confirm that AMH and inhibin B are markers of Sertoli cell function. Sperm DNA damage is moderately increased in male factor infertility, and is negatively associated with sperm motility. A negative association between antioxidant activity and sperm concentration suggests that even minimal oxidative stress may influence sperm concentration. **However, there was no significant relationship between hormone concentrations, sperm DNA damage and total antioxidant capacity, suggesting other mechanisms for sperm dysfunction.** (Appasamy et al, 2007)

Verit et al studies found that the most common cause of male infertility is idiopathic. Standard investigations reveal no abnormality in such cases. The aim of the study was to investigate the levels of sperm DNA damage and seminal oxidative stress and their relationships with idiopathic infertility. The study included 30 normozoospermic infertile men seeking infertility treatment and 20 fertile donors. Semen analysis was performed according to the World Health Organization guidelines. Sperm DNA damage was assessed by alkaline single cell gel electrophoresis (comet assay) after preparation with two-step discontinuous Percoll gradient. Seminal oxidative stress was measured by a novel automated method. DNA damage score, total antioxidant status (TAS), total oxidant status (TOS) and oxidative stress index (OSI) were not different in idiopathic infertile men compared with controls. **No correlations were also found between DNA damage score and TAS, TOS levels and OSI in idiopathic infertile group. We did not find any relationship between sperm DNA damage and oxidative stress in normozoospermic infertile men.** Verit et al think that **the pathophysiology of idiopathic infertility cannot be explained by sperm DNA damage or seminal oxidative stress.** (Verit et at, 2006)

Similarly, some studies have found that **seminal antioxidant activity is reduced in infertile men with high levels of seminal EMODs** (relative to those with normal levels of EMODs) whereas **others have not shown this.** (Zini et al, 1993) (Lewis et al, 1995) (Smith et al, 1996) (Sanocka et al, 1996)

To date, there are no studies to indicate a relationship between systemic antioxidant or vitamin deficiency and male infertility. Silver et al, 2005 evaluated a cohort of fertile men and did not identify any relationships between dietary antioxidant intake (vitamins C, E or ß-carotene) and sperm DNA

damage. (Silver et al, 2005). I believe that this sums it up, in that there is no relationship between antioxidant supplement intake and prevention of DNA damage.

Effect of antioxidant intake on sperm chromatin stability in healthy non-smoking men (Silver et al, 2005) (#87)

Silver et al stated that oxidative stress is detrimental to sperm function and a significant factor in the etiology of male infertility. This report examines the association between dietary and supplementary intake of the antioxidants vitamin C, vitamin E, and beta-carotene and sperm chromatin integrity. **Eighty-seven healthy male volunteers** donated semen samples, completed food-frequency questionnaires, and provided information about their socio-demographic characteristics, medical and reproductive histories, and lifestyle habits. Sperm chromatin integrity was measured using the **DNA fragmentation index (DFI)** and related parameters, obtained from the sperm chromatin structure assay (SCSA). SCSA measures the susceptibility of sperm DNA to acid-induced denaturation in situ. After adjusting for age and duration of abstinence, **there was no dose-response association between any DNA fragmentation index (DFI) outcome and any antioxidant intake measure.** Non-dose-related associations were found between beta-carotene intake and both the standard deviation of DFI (SD DFI) and the percent of immature sperm. Participants with moderate, but not high, beta-carotene intake had an increase in SD DFI compared with participants with low intake (adjusted means 206.7 and 180.5, respectively; P = .03), as well as an increase in the percentage of immature sperm (adjusted means 6.9% and 5.0%, respectively; P = .04). If antioxidant intake in the range studied is indeed beneficial for fertility in healthy men, it does not appear to be mediated through the integrity of sperm chromatin. (Silver et al, 2005)

Nonetheless, it is possible that a subset of infertile men may be at risk for antioxidant deficiency, particularly, vitamin C deficiency. (Hampl et al, 2004)

Moreover, infertile men with specific lifestyles may also be at risk for antioxidant or vitamin deficiency (e.g. smoking, increased alcohol intake, dieting). (Jacob, 1990) (Ryle, Thompson, 1984)

The association of folate, zinc and antioxidant intake with sperm aneuploidy in healthy non-smoking men (Young et al, 2008) (#89)

Little is known about the effect of paternal nutrition on aneuploidy in sperm. We investigated the association of normal dietary and supplement intake of folate, zinc and antioxidants (vitamin C, vitamin E and beta-carotene) with the frequency of aneuploidy in human sperm. METHODS: Sperm samples from **89 healthy, non-smoking men** from a non-clinical setting were analyzed for aneuploidy using fluorescent in situ hybridization with probes for chromosomes X, Y and 21. Daily total intake (diet and supplements) for zinc, folate, vitamin C, vitamin E and beta-carotene was derived from a food frequency questionnaire. Potential confounders were obtained from a self-administered questionnaire. RESULTS: After adjusting for covariates, men with high folate intake (>75th percentile) had lower frequencies of sperm with disomies X, 21, sex nullisomy, and a lower aggregate measure of sperm aneuploidy (P <or= 0.04) compared with men with lower intake. In adjusted continuous analyses, total folate intake was inversely associated with aggregate sperm aneuploidy (-3.6% change/100 microg folate; 95% CI: -6.3, -0. 8) and results were similar for disomies X, 21 and sex nullisomy. **No consistent associations were found between antioxidant or zinc intakes and sperm aneuploidy.** CONCLUSIONS: Men with high folate intake had lower overall frequencies of several types of aneuploid sperm. (Young et al, 2008)

A randomized control trial examining the effect of an antioxidant (Menevit) on pregnancy outcome during IVF-ICSI treatment (Tremellen et al, 2007) (#60 couples)

Evidence has accumulated supporting the role of reactive oxygen species (ROS) in the pathogenesis of sperm dysfunction among men with infertility. Damage to sperm DNA by ROS can lead to failure of conception, miscarriage or potentially even childhood cancer. The objective of this study was to examine the effect of male antioxidant treatment on embryo quality and pregnancy outcome during in vitro fertilisation-intracytoplasmic sperm injection (IVF-ICSI) treatment. METHODS: Sixty couples with severe male factor infertility were enrolled in a prospective randomized double-blind placebo-controlled trial. Male participants were randomly assigned to take either one capsule per day of the Menevit antioxidant or an identical in appearance placebo for three months prior to their partner's IVF cycle. The primary outcome was cleavage stage embryo quality and the secondary outcomes were oocyte fertilization rate, pregnancy rates and treatment side-effects. Approval by the local Human Research Ethics Committee was obtained prior to the commencement of this study. RESULTS: The antioxidant group recorded a statistically significant improvement in viable pregnancy rate (38.5% of transferred embryos resulting in a viable fetus at 13 weeks gestation) compared to the control group (16% viable pregnancy). No significant changes in oocyte fertilization rate or embryo quality were detected between the antioxidant and the placebo groups. *Side-effects on the Menevit antioxidant were rare (8%) and mild in nature.* CONCLUSIONS: The Menevit antioxidant appears to be a useful ancillary treatment that significantly improves pregnancy rates in couples undergoing IVF-ICSI treatment for severe male factor infertility. (Tremellen et al, 2007)

Dietary antioxidant supplements and sperm DNA damage

In order to be active, a dietary antioxidant should be effectively absorbed and concentrated in reproductive tract organs. The antioxidant should also replete a deficiency (in the testis, epididymis or semen) and play a role in reproductive function. The antioxidant must either improve spermatogenesis and/or epididymal function, ultimately, resulting in improved sperm function and chromatin compaction and integrity. Alternatively, the antioxidant should enhance semen antioxidant capacity in order to reduce oxidative DNA damage. **The overall data does not support these notions.**

There are a small number of reports on the effects of dietary antioxidant supplementation on sperm DNA integrity. In general, these are small studies that do not evaluate the mechanism of action of antioxidants: the only endpoint that is measured is the integrity of the sperm DNA or pregnancy rate. Moreover, most studies evaluate the effects of a short treatment course (with no long-term follow-up), are **not randomized and fail to include a placebo-control group.**

Most of these clinical studies have evaluated men with high levels of sperm DNA damage. **In these men, treatment with antioxidant supplements is generally associated with reduced levels of sperm DNA integrity and/or improved fertility potential.** (Greco et al, 2005) (Greco, Iacobelli et al, 2005) (Menezo et al, 2007) (Tremellen et al, 2007) (Gil-Villa et al, 2008) (Piomboni et al, 2008)

In 1991, Fraga et al. demonstrated that dietary vitamin C increases semen vitamin C levels and improves sperm DNA integrity (lowers DNA oxidation levels) in men with a vitamin C deficiency (on a vitamin C depleted diet). **More recent studies of infertile men with high levels of sperm DNA damage (2** randomized controlled and 3 uncontrolled trials) have shown that antioxidant therapy is effective in improving sperm DNA integrity or pregnancy rates.

In men with unselected infertility, the effect of dietary antioxidants on sperm DNA integrity is equivocal with one of two controlled trials showing a benefit of antioxidants on sperm DNA integrity.

In vitro antioxidants and sperm DNA damage

Several studies have examined the role of in vitro antioxidant supplementation in protecting the sperm DNA from oxidative damage. This is clinically relevant as sperm washing is routinely performed prior to ARTs (e.g. intrauterine insemination and in vitro fertilization) and the process may result in injury to the sperm DNA, particularly, as spermatozoa are now vulnerable to oxidative stress because **seminal plasma (rich in antioxidants)** has been removed in the process. (Twigg et al, 1998)

However, it is important to note that subpopulations of spermatozoa will exhibit variable susceptibility to oxidative stress: **the DNA of normal spermatozoa is reportedly less susceptible to gentle processing techniques than is the DNA of abnormal or immature spermatozoa.** (Muratori et al, 2000) (Said et al, 2005)

The studies on in vitro antioxidant supplementation have looked at the role of antioxidants in protecting sperm from exogenous and endogenous EMODs, and, from the effects of semen processing and cryopreservation. **Antioxidants (e.g. vitamins C and E, catalase, glutathione) have been shown quite clearly to protect sperm DNA from the effects of exogenous EMODs.** (Lopes et al, 1998) (Potts et al, 2004) ((Russo et al, 2006)

This is of clinical relevance as many of the semen samples contain leukocytes and these cells have the potential to generate exogenous EMODs. **In contrast, antioxidants appear to be of limited value in protecting the DNA of normal spermatozoa from endogenous EMOD production (e.g. NADPH-induced or centrifugation-induced).** (Twigg et al, 1998) (Cemeli et al, 2004) (Dobrzynska et al, 2004) (Anderson et al, 2003)

In samples with poor morphology and poor sperm chromatin compaction, antioxidants may protect the sperm DNA from endogenous EMOD production, as these samples are more vulnerable to oxidative stress. (Muratori et al, 2000) (Said et al, 2005)

In general, antioxidants appear to be of limited value in protecting sperm DNA from gentle semen processing (e.g. incubation or density-gradient centrifugation). (Chi et al, 2008) (Donnelley et al, 1999) (Hughes et al, 1998) (Donnelly et al, 2000)

In some cases, antioxidant supplementation in vitro (e.g. combination of vitamins C and E) may cause sperm DNA damage. (Donnelly et al, 1999) (Hughes et al, 1998)

The effect of ascorbate and alpha-tocopherol supplementation in vitro on DNA integrity and hydrogen peroxide-induced DNA damage in human spermatozoa (Donnelly et al, 1999) (#) The aim of this study was to determine the effects of supplementation with ascorbate and alpha-tocopherol, both singly and in combination, during sperm preparation on subsequent sperm DNA integrity, induced DNA damage and reactive oxygen species (ROS) generation. Semen samples with normozoospermic and asthenozoospermic profiles (n = 15 for each control and antioxidant group) were prepared by Percoll density centrifugation (95.0-47.5%) where the medium had been supplemented with these antioxidants to a number of different concentrations, all within physiological levels. Controls were included which had no ascorbate or alpha-tocopherol added. DNA damage was induced using hydrogen peroxide ($H(2)O(2)$) and DNA integrity was determined using a modified alkaline single cell gel electrophoresis (Comet) assay, while ROS generation was measured using chemiluminescence. Addition of ascorbate to sperm preparation medium did not affect baseline DNA integrity but did provide sperm with complete protection against $H(2)O(2)$-induced DNA damage. Generation of $H(2)O(2)$-induced ROS was also significantly reduced after treatment with ascorbate, although baseline levels were unaffected by this antioxidant. Supplementation of sperm preparation medium with alpha-tocopherol did not influence baseline DNA integrity but provided sperm with dose-dependent protection against $H(2)O(2)$-induced DNA damage. Generation of $H(2)O(2)$-induced ROS was significantly reduced after treatment with alpha-tocopherol, although baseline ROS levels were unaffected by this antioxidant. *Addition of both ascorbate and alpha-tocopherol in combination to sperm preparation medium actually induced DNA damage and intensified the damage induced by H(2)O(2)*, however, H(2)O(2)-induced ROS production was significantly reduced in a dose-dependent manner by supplementation with both vitamins. (Donnelly et al, 1999)

Glutathione and hypotaurine in vitro: effects on human sperm motility, DNA integrity and production of reactive oxygen species (Donnelly et al, 2000)

Sperm DNA integrity is of paramount importance for the accurate conveyance of genetic material. DNA damage may be a major contributory factor in male infertility as DNA from sperm of infertile men has been found to be more susceptible to induced DNA damage in vitro than DNA from fertile men. Reactive oxygen species (ROS) are a significant source of DNA damage and human sperm are extremely sensitive to ROS attack due to their high content of polyunsaturated fatty acids and lack of capacity for DNA repair. Seminal plasma, which contains a wealth of antioxidants, provides sperm with crucial protection against oxidative insult. However, during preparation for use in assisted conception techniques, sperm are separated from seminal plasma and deprived of that essential protection. The aim of this study was to determine the effects of supplementation with glutathione and hypotaurine during sperm preparation on subsequent sperm motility, DNA integrity, induced DNA damage and ROS generation. Semen samples (n = 45) were divided into aliquots and prepared by Percoll density centrifugation (95.0-47.5%) using medium which had been supplemented with these antioxidants to a number of different concentrations all within physiological levels. Control aliquots were included which had no glutathione or hypotaurine added. Sperm motility was determined using computer-assisted semen analysis. DNA damage was induced using H(2)O(2) and DNA integrity was determined using a modified alkaline single cell gel electrophoresis (Comet) assay, while ROS generation was measured using chemiluminescence. **Addition of glutathione and hypotaurine, either singly or in combination, to sperm preparation medium had no significant effect on sperm progressive motility or baseline DNA integrity.** Despite this, sperm were still afforded significant protection against H(2)O(2)-induced damage and ROS generation. (Donnelly et al, 2000)

The one study evaluating the effects of sperm cryopreservation suggests that antioxidants (vitamin E) do not protect sperm DNA in this setting. (Taylor et al, 2009)

Summary

In summary, the data suggest that ROS appear to play an important role in the generation of sperm DNA damage. Although in vitro studies have demonstrated a beneficial effect of antioxidant supplements in protecting sperm DNA from exogenous oxidants, **the effect of these antioxidants in protecting sperm from endogenous EMODs, gentle sperm processing and cryopreservation has not been established.** The data suggest that dietary antioxidants may be beneficial in reducing sperm DNA damage, particularly, in men with high levels of DNA fragmentation. **However, the mechanism of action of dietary antioxidants has not been established and most of the clinical studies are small.** (Zini et al, 2009)

CHAPTER TWENTY TWO

Role of antioxidants in treatment of male infertility: an overview of the literature (Agarwal et al, 2004)

Seminal oxidative stress in the male reproductive tract is known to result in peroxidative damage of the sperm plasma membrane and loss of its DNA integrity. Normally, a balance exists between concentrations of reactive oxygen species and antioxidant scavenging systems. One of the rational strategies to counteract the oxidative stress is to increase the scavenging capacity of seminal plasma. Numerous studies have evaluated the efficacy of antioxidants in male infertility. In this review, the results of different studies conducted have been analyzed, and the evidence available to date is provided. **It was found that although many clinical trials have demonstrated the beneficial effects of antioxidants in selected cases of male infertility, some studies failed to demonstrate the same benefit. The majority of the studies suffer from a lack of placebo-controlled, double-blind design, making it difficult to reach a definite conclusion.** In addition, investigators have used different antioxidants in different combinations and dosages for varying durations. Pregnancy, the most relevant outcome parameter of fertility, was reported in only a few studies. Most studies failed to examine the effect of antioxidants on a specific group of infertile patients with high oxidative stress. Multicenter, double-blind studies with statistically accepted sample size are still needed to provide conclusive evidence on the benefit of antioxidants as a treatment modality for patients with male infertility. (Agarwal et al, 2004)

Impacts of oxidative stress and antioxidants on semen functions

Oxidative stress (OS) has been considered a major contributory factor to the infertility. Oxidative stress is the result of imbalance between the reactive oxygen species (ROS) and antioxidants in the body which can lead to sperm damage, deformity, and eventually male infertility. Although high concentrations of the ROS cause sperm pathology (ATP depletion) leading to insufficient axonemal phosphorylation, lipid peroxidation, and loss of motility and viability but, **many evidences demonstrate that low and controlled concentrations of these ROS play an important role in sperm physiological processes such as capacitation, acrosome reaction, and signaling processes to ensure fertilization.** The supplementation of a cryopreservation extender with antioxidant has been shown to provide a cryoprotective effect on mammalian sperm quality. This paper reviews the impacts of oxidative stress and reactive oxygen species on spermatozoa functions, causes of ROS generation, and antioxidative strategies to reduce OS. In addition, we also highlight the emerging concept of utilizing OS as a tool of contraception. (Bansal, Bilaspuri, 2010)

It is very important to identify the factors/conditions which affect normal sperm functions. **Among various causes, oxidative stress (OS) has been attributed to affect the fertility status and physiology of spermatozoa.** (Agarwal et al, 2008)

The term oxidative stress is generally applied when oxidants outnumber antioxidants. (du Plessis et al, 2008)

The imbalance between the production of reactive oxygen species (ROS) and a biological systems ability to readily detoxify the reactive intermediates or easily repair the resulting damage is known as oxidative stress. (Agarwal et al, 2003)

The main destructive aspects of oxidative stress are the production of ROS, which include free radicals and peroxides. (Valko et al, 2005)

The production of EMODs by sperm is a normal physiological process, but an imbalance between ROS generation and scavenging activity is detrimental to the sperm and associated with male infertility. (Sharma, Agarwal, 1996)

Physiological levels of EMODs influence and mediate the gametes. (Gagnon et al, 1991) (Aitken, 1997) (Attaran et al, 2000) **and crucial reproduc-**

tive processes, such as sperm-oocyte interactions (de Lamirande et al, 1997), implantation and early embryo development. (Sakkas, 1998)

Against ROS attack, sperm cells are well equipped with a powerful defense system of antioxidants. Antioxidants are the main defense factors against oxidative stress induced by free radicals.

Free radicals are short lived reactive chemical intermediates, which contain one or more unpaired electrons. (Kefer et al, 2009) (Sanocka, Kurpisz, 2004)

They induce cellular damages when they pass this unpaired electron onto nearby cellular structures, resulting in oxidation of cell membrane lipids, amino acids in proteins or within nucleic acids.

Free radicals are also known as a necessary evil for intracellular signaling involved in the normal process of cell proliferation, differentiation, and migration. (Agarwal et al, 2004) (Rhee, 2006) (Ford, 2001)

In the reproductive tract, free radicals also play a dual role and can modulate various reproductive functions. (du Plessis et al, 2008)

Excess of free radicals generation frequently involves an error in spermiogenesis resulting in the release of spermatozoa from the germinal epithelium exhibiting abnormally high levels of cytoplasmic retention. (Sanocka, Kurpisz, 2004)

EMODs are formed as necessary by-products during the normal enzymatic reactions of inter- and intracellular signaling. Mammalian spermatozoa represent a growing list of cell types that exhibit a capacity to generate ROS when incubated under aerobic conditions, such as, hydrogen peroxide (H_2O_2), the superoxide anion ($^\bullet O_2^-$), the hydroxyl radical ($OH_\bullet$), and hypochlorite radical ($OHCl_\bullet$). Due to their highly reactive nature, ROS can combine readily with other molecules, directly causing oxidation that can lead to structural and functional changes and result in cellular damage. (Guerin et al, 2001) (de Lamirande, Gagnon, 1995) (Agarwal, Gupta, et al, 2005)

EMODs represent a broad category of molecules that indicate the collection of radicals (hydroxyl ion, superoxide, nitric oxide, peroxyl, etc.) and non-radicals (ozone, single oxygen, lipid peroxides, hydrogen peroxide) and oxygen derivatives. (Agarwal, Prabakaran, 2005)

Reactive nitrogen species (nitrous oxide, peroxynitrite, nitroxyl ion, etc.) are free nitrogen radicals and considered a subclass of ROS. (Sikka, 2001) (Darley-Usmar et al, 1995)

Nitric oxide (NO) has been shown to have detrimental effects on normal sperm functions inhibiting both motility and sperm competence for zona binding. (Agarwal et al, 2008)

In males, two ROS (EMOD) generating systems are possibly involved, a hypothetical NADH oxidase at the level of sperm membrane and low sperm diphorase (mitochondrial NADH-dependent oxidoreductase). In bovine semen, ROS are generated primarily by dead spermatozoa via an aromatic amino acid oxidase catalyzed reaction.

Leukocytes and immature spermatozoa are the two main sources of EMODs. (Garrido et al, 2004)

Leukocytes particularly neutrophils and macrophages have been associated with excessive EMOD production and they ultimately cause sperm dysfunction. (Aitken et al, 1995) (Shalika et al, 1996) (Aitken, Fisher, et al, 1997) (Hendin et al, 1999) (Pasqualotto et al, 2000) (Sharma et al, 2001) (Saleh et al, 2002)

Two of the main factors contributing to ROS accumulation *in vitro* are the absence of endogenous defense mechanism and second exposure of gametes and embryos to various manipulation techniques as well as environment that can lead to generation of oxidative stress.

Levels of EMODs may rarely fluctuate within a fertile individual, but, do not affect sperm concentration and motility. This may be due to the presence of adequate antioxidant defense mechanisms in the healthy individuals. The fluctuations in ROS levels might be due to transient subclinical infection and transient abnormalities in spermatogenesis such as, retention of cytoplasm or periodic presence of abnormal spermatozoa in semen.

The production of EMODs is a normal physiological process but an imbalance between ROS generation and scavenging activity is detrimental to the sperm and associated with male infertility.

EMODs generated by spermatozoa play an important role in normal physiological processes such as, sperm capacitation, acrosome reaction, mainte-

nance of fertilizing ability, and stabilization of the mitochondrial capsule in the mid-piece in bovine. (Agarwal et al, 2008) (Goncalves et al, 2010) (Desai et al, 2009)

Controlled generation of ROS may function as signaling molecules (second messengers) in many different cell types; they are important mediators of sperm functions. **Evidences have been reported that especially superoxide anion ($^.O_2$) is required for the late stage of embryo development such as, two germ cell layers and egg cylinder.** (Kodama et al, 1996)

Although a significant negative correlation between ROS and IVF fertilization rate has been found, yet, **controlled generation of ROS has shown to be essential for the development of capacitation and hyperactivation, the two processes of sperm that are necessary to ensure fertilization.** (de Lamirande, Gagnon, 1993)

In vivo physiological concentrations of ROS are involved in providing membrane fluidity, maintaining the fertilizing ability and acrosome reaction of sperm. (Bucak et al, 2010)

The maintenance of a suitable ROS level is, therefore, essential for adequate sperm functionality. ROS cause adverse effects on the sperm plasma membrane, DNA, and physiological processes, thereby, affecting the quality of spermatozoa. **The axosome and associated dense fibers of the mid-piece in sperm are covered by mitochondria that generate energy from intracellular stores of ATP depletion.** (Bucak et al, 2008)

Excessive ROS impairs motility and capacity of fertilization. Additionally, cold shock arising from other stress plays an important role in the molding of membranes by determining their sol gel balance and the dynamic status that affects the fusion of the plasma membrane of the male and female gametes. (Bucak et al, 2007)

The assumption that ROS can influence male fertility has received substantial scientific support.

Mammalian spermatozoal membranes are rich in polyunsaturated fatty acids (PUFAs) and are sensitive to oxygen-induced damage mediated by lipid peroxidation, and, thus are sensitive to ROS attack which results in decreased sperm motility, presumably by a rapid loss of intracellular ATP leading to axonemal damage, decreased sperm viability, and increased mid-piece sperm morphological defects with deleterious effects on sperm capacitation and acrosome reaction. (Bansal, Bilaspuri, 2007)

Thus, EMODs (ROS) are independent markers of male factor infertility.

Measurement of MDA and TBA

Malondialdehyde (MDA) is an end product of LPO which is measured through thiobarbituric acid (TBA) assay. TBA reactive substances (TBARS) are mainly formed during the determination of LPO *in vitro*. **In many studies, TBARS level, as an indicator of LPO, was increased in frozen thawed bull sperm, but, not in cooled sperm.** (Chatterjee, Gagnon, 2001)

Malondialdehyde (MDA) levels do not differ in fresh and frozen semen in normal men. (Wang et al, 1997)

In bull semen, spontaneous LPO is measured by the endogenous lipid peroxides.

Antioxidants

Spermatozoa are protected by various antioxidants and antioxidant enzymes in the seminal plasma or in spermatozoa itself to prevent oxidative damage. An antioxidant that reduces oxidative stress and improves sperm motility could be useful in the management of male infertility. **Antioxidants are the agents, which break the oxidative chain reaction, thereby, reduce the oxidative stress).** (Miller et al, 1993) (Kumar, Mahmood, 2001)

Vitamin E (antioxidant) may directly quench the free radicals such as peroxyl and alkoxyl ($ROO_.$) generated during ferrous ascorbate-induced LPO, thus it is suggested as major chain breaking antioxidant. Antioxidants, in general, are the compounds and reactions which dispose, scavenge, and suppress the formation of ROS, or oppose their actions. Mn^{2+} enhances sperm motility, viability, capacitation and acrosome reaction by decreasing the oxidative stress. Extracellular addition of Mn^{2+} ions also enhances the level of cAMP by stimulating Ca^{2+} or Mg^{2+} ATPase which leads to activation of calcium channel opening, thereby depositing more Ca_i^{2+}. Thus, Mn^{2+} promotes the acrosome reaction.

Thiol groups also play an important role in detoxification and antioxidation of ROS, besides maintaining the intracellular redox status. These groups serve as defense mechanisms of sperm cells to fight against oxidative stress. A variety of biological and chemical antioxidants that attack ROS and LPO are presently under investigation.

Recent studies demonstrate that **supplementation of cryopreservation extenders with antioxidants has been shown to provide a cryoprotective effect on bull, ram, goat, boar, canine, and human sperm quality, thus improving semen parameters, for example, sperm motility, membrane integrity after thawing.** (Bucak et al, 2010)

Supplementation with these antioxidants prior to the cryopreservation process may be recommended to facilitate the enhancement of sperm cryopreservation technique for the goat breeding industry. Supplementation with antioxidants during IVF procedures impaired sperm quality, normal pronuclear formation, and embryo development to the blastocyst stage.

Enzymatic Antioxidants

Enzymatic antioxidants are also known as natural antioxidants; they neutralize excess ROS and prevent it from damaging the cellular structure. Enzymatic antioxidants are composed of superoxide dismutase (SOD), catalase, glutathione peroxidase (GPx), and glutathione reductase (GR) which also causes reduction of hydrogen peroxides to water and alcohol. SOD spontaneously dismutase superoxide anion $(O_2^{-\bullet})$ to form O_2 and H_2O_2 while catalase converts H_2O_2 to O_2 and H_2O.

SOD protects spermatozoa against spontaneous O_2 toxicity and LPO. (Sikka, 1996)

SOD and catalase also remove $O_2^{-\bullet}$ generated by NADPH oxidase in neutrophils and play a major role in decreasing LPO and protecting spermatozoa against oxidative damage. (Sikka, 1996)

Catalase presence in sperm has been demonstrated for ram and cattle and it has a potential role in ageing process and control of oxidative stress in cells, mainly resulting from H_2O_2. (Bucak et al, 2007)

Nonenzymatic Antioxidants

Nonenzymatic antioxidants are also known as synthetic antioxidants or dietary supplements. The body's complex antioxidant system is influenced by dietary intake of antioxidants, vitamins, and minerals such as vitamin C, vitamin E, zinc, taurine, hypotaurine, and glutathione. (Agarwal et al, 2005)

Glutathione is a molecule found at mM level in a number of cells, able to react with many ROS directly. (Bucak et al, 2008)

GSH is also a cofactor for GSHPx that catalyzes the reduction of **toxic H_2O_2** and other hydroperoxides, protecting the mammalian cells from oxidative stress. (Bucak et al, 2008)

Glutamine (5 mM) has been provided a cryoprotective effect by improving post thaw motility, membrane integrity, and catalase enzyme activity in ram semen.

Supplementation of inositol in the extender can improve the motility of frozen thawed bull sperm. Inositol has cryoprotective and antioxidative properties resulting in higher antioxidant GSH activity, acrosome integrity, and intact morphological rates.

Cysteine is a low-molecular weight amino acid containing thiol; it is a precursor of intracellular glutathione. It has been shown to penetrate the cell membrane easily, enhancing the intracellular GSH biosynthesis both *in vivo* and *in vitro* and protecting the membrane lipids and proteins due to indirect radical scavenging properties. **It is also thought that GSH synthesis under *in vitro* conditions may be impaired because of deficiency of cysteine in the media, due to its high instability and auto-oxidation to cysteine.** (Bucak et al, 2008)

Cysteine has cryoprotective effect on the functional integrity of axosome and mitochondria improving post thawed sperm motility. It has been proved that thiols such as glutathione and cysteine prevented the loss of sperm motility in frozen thawed bull semen. Cysteine has been shown to prevent the loss in motility of frozen thawed bull, ram, and goat semen and to improve viability, the chromatin structure, and membrane integrity of boar sperm during liquid preservation. Cysteine has improved the porcine oocytes maturation and fertilization *in vitro*.

Trehalose or taurine, a sulfonic amino acid, acts as nonenzymatic scavenger that plays an important role in the protection of spermatozoa against ROS, in case of exposure to aerobic conditions and the freezing—thawing process. A non-permanent disaccharide has a protective action related both to osmotic effect and specific interactions with membrane phospholipids, rendering hypertonic media, causing cellular osmotic dehydration before freezing and then decreasing the amount of cell injury by its crystallization. Trehalose performs better cryoprotection post thaw fertilizing ability in ram, bull, and mouse sperm due to diminished death and damage of sperm. A recent study has demonstrated that antioxidant capacity of trehalose is observed upon the performance of incubation at 37°C for 3 h and no difference is obtained at 0 h post thawing of ram semen. Tuarine displayed antioxidative properties by elevating catalase level in close association with superoxide dismutase concentration in ram, rabbit, and bull spermatozoa.

Hyaluronan, an essential component of the extracellular matrix and nonsulfated glycosaminoglycan, is involved in important physiological functions such as motility, capacitation of spermatozoa and preserve post thaw spermatozoa viability, and *in vitro* membrane stability. Hyaluronan improves sperm motility, viability and membrane integrity after freezing and thawing procedure and decrease polyspermy with declining motility in humans and boars.

Bovine serum albumin (BSA) is known to eliminate free radicals generated by oxidative stress and protect membrane integrity of sperm cells from heat shock during freezing-thawing of canine semen.

Carotenoids such as beta-carotene and lycopene are also important components of antioxidant defense. Beta carotenes protect the plasma membrane against LPO in rat.

Addition of antioxidants vitamin E, butylated hydroxytoluene (BHT), and Tempo to extended turkey semen improves sperm survival and membrane integrity and reduces the loss of motility after 48 h of storage.

Since long it has been known that supplementation of culture media with antioxidants such as, ROS scavengers, disulfide reducing, or divalent chelators prolongs the motility of reactivated bull spermatozoa after freezing and thawing. (Tarin et al, 1998)

It has been suggested that antioxidant therapy appears to be efficient not only *in vitro* but also *in vivo*. (Tarin et al, 1998)

Numerous antioxidants have proven beneficial in protecting damaging effects of ROS on sperm movement and against oxidative damage. (Yousef et al, 2003)

Lipid peroxidation induced by H_2O_2 not only disrupts sperm motility, but, also impairs all the sperm functions which are dependent on the integrity of plasma membrane, including sperm-oocyte fusion and ability to undergo acrosomal exocytose. Such findings have raised the possibility that hydrogen peroxide or reagents producing them on contact with spermatozoa might be an effective way of contraception. (Bansal, Bilaspuri, 2010)

Antioxidant therapy in male infertility: fact or fiction?

Infertile men have higher levels of semen reactive oxygen species (ROS, EMODs) than do fertile men. High levels of semen ROS can cause sperm dysfunction, sperm DNA damage and reduced male reproductive potential. This observation has led clinicians to treat infertile men with antioxidant supplements. The purpose of this article is to discuss the rationale for antioxidant therapy in infertile men and to evaluate the data on the efficacy of dietary and in vitro antioxidant preparations on sperm function and DNA damage. To date, most clinical studies suggest that dietary antioxidant supplements are beneficial in terms of improving sperm function and DNA integrity. **However, the exact mechanism of action of dietary antioxidants and the optimal dietary supplement have not been established. Moreover, most of the clinical studies are small and few have evaluated pregnancy rates.** A beneficial effect of in vitro antioxidant supplements in protecting spermatozoa from exogenous oxidants has been demonstrated in most studies; **however, the effect of these antioxidants in protecting sperm from endogenous ROS, gentle sperm processing and cryopreservation has not been established conclusively.** (Zini, Al-Hathal, 2011)

Sperm, Reactive Oxygen Species (ROS) and Anti-Oxidants

Reactive oxygen species (ROS) are molecules that are highly disruptive to cellular function, in general, and have been shown to play a role in male factor infertility. ROS have free radicals, which are unpaired electrons which tend to bind other molecules and alter them. The ROS of primary interest are the superoxide anion ($\cdot O_2^-$), hydroxyl radical ($\cdot OH$), and hypochlorite radical ($\cdot OHCl$). **These damage cells of all types and may play a role in as much as 40% of male factor infertility.** (Sharma, Agarwal, 1996)

The sperm cell is highly susceptible to damage by these highly reactive molecules because of its unique structure. **The spermatozoon has a unique lipid membrane covering its head** that is involved with attachment to the egg zona pellucida as well as important changes that occur with the capacitation reaction. The sperm head also contains important acrosome enzymes as well as the chromosomes that will eventually fuse with the maternal chromosomes. **The mid-piece of the sperm generates the power to propel the tail by generating energy using its mitochondria.** These mitochondria generate reactive oxygen molecules and are the aerobic source of cell energy.

Thus, **sperm acquire motility because of oxidative metabolism in their mitochondria. Obviously, antioxidants may negatively interfere with this oxidative process. (RMH)**

Semen also contains white blood cells, a very important source of ROS. The discussion below will review what ROS are and how they are generated. Studies will be reviewed that show an association with male factor infertility will be discussed as well as how the ROS affect the sperm components. Finally, studies using anti-oxidants will be reviewed as they relate to male factor infertility.

Sperm are produced in the testes and spend approximately 10 days in the epididymis where they undergo important maturation stages. **It is in the epididymis that oxidative damage may occur to the sperm.** (Vernet et al, 2004)

Sperm have polyunsaturated fatty acids, making up approximately 40 % of the lipids in the sperm head, which are important for membrane fluidity, sperm motility, capacitation, and sperm binding to the egg zona pellucida. **These polyunsaturated fatty acids are extremely susceptible to oxidative damage.** 'Oxidative Stress' is an imbalance between the ROS generating factors and ROS scavenging systems.

It is somewhat ironic that sperm may produce ROS when they utilize their oxidative metabolism to provide movement and so may damage them selves in addition to playing a role in normal sperm function such as hyperactivation, capacitation, acrosome reaction, oocyte penetration, and signal transduction (via tyrosine phosphorylase).

The internal sources of sperm ROS are the mitochondria (primary) which generate hydrogen peroxide (H2O2) and the sperm plasma membrane NADPH oxidase system. (Agarwal et al, 2003)

External sources of ROS include white blood cells in the -lymphocytesbsemen. These produce H2O2 and Oxygen (O2). The phagocytes and produce −O2 which appear to use NADPH oxidase like enzymes.

Low levels of ROS may be generated by other cells in the male reproductive tract including endothelial cells, fibroblasts, mesangial cells, and vascular smooth muscle cells. (Vernet et al, 2004)

As you can see, overproduction could come from several sources. Infection of the prostate, i.e. prostatitis, is associated with decreased sperm motility, anti-sperm antibodies, and oxidative stress. ROS may be increased with certain medications, radiation, pollutants and in patients with spinal cord injuries. (Potts, Pasaqualotto, 2003)

The sperm scavengers in seminal plasma include vitamin E (α-tocopherol), vitamin C (ascorbic acid), uric acid, glutathione, taurine, hypotaurine, and albumin. (Sharma, Agarwal, 1996)

A group of enzymes (Potts, Pasaqualotto, 2003) also help to scavenge oxygen radicals throughout the male reproductive tract (glutathione peroxidase, catalase, indolamine dioxygenase, and superoxide dismutase)

It is important to realize that the body has redundant systems to remove these potentially toxic compounds. When these systems fail, it is possible that oxidative stress may occur leading to sperm damage. Experiments where sperm were exposed to artificially produced ROS showed DNA damage and programmed cell death. (Agarwal et al, 2003) (Sonmez et al, 2005) showed that vitamin C increased the epididymal sperm concentration and plasma testosterone levels in male rats that had their diets supplemented.

Mishra and Acharya (Mishra, Acharya, 2004) showed that Vitamin C and E were protective to the experimental damage caused be lead exposure in experiments where mice were exposed to doses of lead that would normally impair spermatogenesis.

In an additional experimental model, (Strzezek et al, 2004) showed that a dietary supplement of polyunsaturated fatty acids and antioxidants had beneficial effects on boar sperm.

Similar positive effects were noted by Audet et al, (Audet et al, 2004) in boars where sperm motility was increased with the vitamin supplements.

Several studies addressed antioxidant use humans and the effects on sperm. Silver *et al* (Silver et al, 2005) did a questionnaire with 87 healthy male volunteers that had information on antioxidant intake. They failed to show a correlation with their sperm chromatin assay.

However, Greco *et al* (Greco, Romano et al, 2005) had 38 men with documented increased DNA fragmentation and gave them 1 gm of vitamin C and vitamin E daily for 2 months after one failed ICSI attempt and reported improved implantation and pregnancy rates.

The same group (Greco, Iacobelli, et al, 2005) also found that sperm DNA fragmentation was reduced with oral antioxidant treatment.

Another study (Rolf et al, 1999) failed to show a positive effect of antioxidants improving ejaculate parameters (volume, concentration, motility, viability), however this study did not address fertilization or pregnancy rates.

From the above it is possible that oxygen radicals may play a role in male factor infertility. Given the potential positive effects of supplementation, it may be reasonable to include this in our treatment of male patients.

Oxidative stress and antioxidants: exposure and impact on female fertility

(Ruder et al, 2008) http://humupd.oxfordjournals.org/content/14/4/345. full.pdf (see original article for full references)

It is interesting to note that some, but not all, antioxidants have increased Dietary Reference Intakes during pregnancy, as issued by the Food and Nutrition Board, Institute of Medicine (2003). For example, the maternal requirement for vitamin C is increased during pregnancy due to hemodilution and active transfer to the fetus. Certain populations, such as cigarette smokers and heavy users of alcohol, may have further increased vitamin C requirements during pregnancy due to increased lipid peroxidation. In contrast, **sufficient scientific** evidence is not available to support a change in the requirement of vitamin E during pregnancy.

Pregnancy itself may produce OS as a result of increased metabolic activity. Increased plasma thiols in pregnant women (Wisdom et al., 1991) and increased placental lipid peroxides and decreased expression of antioxidants have been reported (Wisdom et al., 1991; Myatt and Cui, 2004). **Substantial increases in OS have been hypothesized to lead to acute pregnancy complications** (Wang et al., 1997) **or spontaneous abortion** (Sane et al., 1991; Vural et al., 2000).

Successful initiation of pregnancy requires the ovulation of a mature oocyte, production of competent sperm, proximity of sperm and oocyte in the reproductive tract, fertilization of the oocyte, transport of the conceptus into the uterus, and implantation of the embryo into a properly prepared, healthy endometrium. A dysfunction in any one of these complex biological steps can cause infertility (Goldman et al., 2000).

Physical activity, in turn, is associated with an increase in ROS (Davies et al., 1982), but appears only to be damaging to tissues when the exercise is exhaustive (Gomez-Cabrera et al., 2003).

Smoking and alcohol are both known to decrease fertility in women (Howe et al., 1985; Hakim et al., 1998), likely through an increase in OS. Cigarette smoke contains a number of ROS (Pryor et al., 1983) and ethanol metabolism generates ROS through the electron transport chain.

It is worth noting that the essentiality of vitamin E for fertility in rodents resulted in its dietary compounds being named 'tocopherol,' the Greek word for 'childbirth' (tocos) and 'to bring forth' (pheros) (Evans, 1963; Gray, 1996).

ROS, antioxidants and reproductive processes in women Oocytes: ovarian germ cells to secondary oocytes

Following hormonal influence at puberty, a number of primary oocytes begin to grow each month. One primary oocyte outgrows the others and resumes meiosis I (MI). Interestingly, **resumption of MI is induced by an increase in ROS and inhibited by antioxidants** (Takami et al., 1999, 2000; Kodaman and Behrman, 2001), **indicating that regulated generation of ROS by the pre-ovulatory follicle is an important promoter of** the ovulatory sequence. However, it has been suggested that cyclical ROS production may, over time, contribute to oophoritis associated with autoimmune premature ovarian failure (Behrman et al., 2001) and exacerbated by diminished antioxidant status.

The contrasting relationship of antioxidants, detrimental for the progression of MI, but beneficial for MII, suggests a complex role for antioxidants and ROS in the ovarian

environment. Such findings, along with others discussed below suggesting a threshold for ROS beneficence where embryo formation is compromised by ROS concentration during IVF treatment, requires an appreciation of ROS as multifunctional agents in which their effects may vary over the continuum of concentration and developmental stages.

Folliculogenesis

Generation of ROS.

Attendant to the increase in steroid hormone production of developing follicles is an increase in the activity of cytochrome P450, which in turn generates ROS such as hydrogen peroxide (H_2O_2) (Ortega-Camarillo et al., 1999). An investigation of ROS regulation by the preovulatory follicle in response to LH indicated that a gonadotrophin-simulated, protein kinase C-activated, NADPH/NADH oxidase-type superoxide generator in the preovulatory follicle exists and may be a regulating factor in ROS production during ovulation (Kodaman and Behrman, 2001).

Hypoxia of the granulosa cells is a normal event during the growth of ovarian follicles (Tropea et al., 2006). Oxygen limitation is known to stimulate follicular angiogenesis, which is important for follicular growth and development. Impairment of angiogenesis within ovarian follicles contributes to follicular atresia (Greenwald and Terranova, 1988). ROS may act as signal transducers (Schroedl et al., 2002) or intracellular messengers (Pearlstein et al., 2002) of the angiogenic response.

Mitochondria are the major consumers of cellular oxygen, thereby providing support to the hypothesis that ROS are involved in intracellular signaling between tissue hypoxia and angiogenic response (Basini et al., 2004).

Folliculogenesis

Follicular atresia and luteal regression. However, the ROS increase can be countered (be it desirable or undesirable) by antioxidant status. Antioxidant properties of E2 were investigated in pig luteal and follicular tissue exposed to in vitro H2O2. **High doses of E2 (_40 pg/ml) protected against apoptosis, but other non-aromatizable steroid hormones (progesterone, testosterone, dihydrotestosterone or cortisol) offered no protection, suggesting that ovarian E2 functions as a ROS scavenger during pregnancy-mediated luteal rescue and folliculogenesis** (Murdoch, 1998).

Interestingly, increased serum GSH reductase (GSHR) was significantly associated with decreased time-to-pregnancy in 83 female participants in a prospective pregnancy study with preconception enrollment recruited from the New York Angler Cohort. **No**

statistically significant associations were found with GSHPx, SOD, catalase or thiobarbituric acid (Jackson et al., 2005a).

Basini et al. (2004) reported that ROS under moderate concentrations plays a role in signal transduction processes involved in growth and protection from apoptosis.

ROS were found to induce a biphasic effect with lower (P , 0.01) and higher concentrations inhibiting proliferation (P , 0.01), suggesting that **controlled**

levels of ROS may be needed to maintain DNA synthesis, T-I cell proliferation, and growth of ovarian mesenchyme.

Corpus lutea function. **The corpus luteum (CL) has a high concentration of antioxidants, particularly beta-carotene, which gives the CL its bright yellow color** (Rodgers et al., 1995). Other carotenoids and vitamins C and E are also present in relatively high concentrations in the CL where they may play an important role in scavenging ROS (Aten et al., 1992, 1994; Matzuk et al., 1998; Behrman et al., 2001). In addition to its antioxidant function, ascorbic acid is a required cofactor in the synthesis of collagen in the luteal extracellular matrix (Luck and Zhao, 1993). **ROS are produced during luteal regression (Behrman et al., 2001), in part though cytochrome P450 enzymes which are necessary for the first step of steroidogenesis** (Rodgers et al., 1995).

Implantation

Nitric oxide (NO), a free radical produced by NO synthases (NOS), functions as an important vasodilator, neurotransmitter, regulator of embryonic development and implantation (Guerin et al., 2001), and may also contribute as an anti-platelet agent during implantation (Schmidt et al., 1992; Cameron and Campbell, 1998). Schmidt et al. (1992) investigated the distribution of NOS in a number of rat organ tissues. **NOS type I (NOS-I) and NADPH-diaphorase (NADPH-d) were found to be highly concentrated in endometrial epithelial cells.** The function of NO in endometrial epithelial cells is not established, but may include regulation of cyclic GMP, which may mediate the estrogen-stimulated rapid uterine secretory response at the implantation site.

In addition, **both ROS and SOD may act as second messengers to regulate endometrial function** (Sugino, 2007).

ROS and TAC were measured by chemiluminescence in the FF of 53 women undergoing IVF by Attaran et al. (2000). **Individuals who became pregnant had significantly higher FF ROS levels than those who did not, although TAC did not differ by pregnancy status.**

Nonetheless, this study suggests **FF ROS, at physiologic concentrations, may be indicative of a metabolically active system and a potential marker of IVF success.**

Wiener-Megnazi et al. (2004) used a thermochemiluminescence (TCL) assay to measure OS in FF samples from 189 women undergoing IVF. **After controlling for age, OS was found to be positively correlated with the number of retrieved mature oocytes (P , 0.0001). These results suggest a beneficial threshold level for OS.** The existence of an acceptable threshold level was also suggested in the evaluation of 208 FF samples from 78 women undergoing controlled ovarian stimulation (Das et al., 2006).

The unique finding of the Das et al. investigation was evidence of a favorable effect of ROS on percent embryo formation up to _100 cps in both Grade II and Grade III oocytes, after which embryo formation declined. Pasqualotto et al. (2004) reported **both lipid peroxidation and TAC to be positively correlated with pregnancy rate, but not fertilization rate.** However, the categorical nature of the correlation precludes the ability to detect differences over the continuum of values.

Impact of ROS on the aging oocyte

Free radical activity of human FF increases with age (Wiener-Megnazi et al., 2004), as does apoptosis of human granulosa and cumulus cells (Sadraie et al., 2000; Moffatt et al., 2002).

Endometriosis.

Furthermore, no correlation between ROS and increasing stage of severity of endometriosis was detected in either the unprocessed or processed (cell-free) peritoneal fluid.

Conclusion

The role of OS in female fertility and subfertility is an area deserving of continued research. The available evidence suggests **gynecologic OS is an important mediator of conception.** In addition, **care must be given to acknowledge potential undesirable effects of excessive vitamin supplementation** (Tarin et al., 1998b).

Free radicals: their beneficial and detrimental effects on sperm function

Free radicals are molecules with one or more unpaired electron(s) commonly found in seminal plasma. Physiologically, **free radicals control sperm maturation, capacitation and hyperactivation, the acrosome reaction, and sperm-oocyte fusion.**

Pathologically, free radicals induce lipid peroxidation, DNA damage and apoptosis of spermatozoa. The present review deals with both the beneficial and detrimental effects of free radicals on sperm function. (Kothari et al, 2010)

Oxygen consumption and ROS production are increased at the time of fertilization and cell cleavage in bovine zygotes

Oxygen consumption is a key indicator of metabolic activity within embryos. **Increased oxidative activity and REDOX changes at the time of fertilization have been suggested to signal Ca(2+) oscillations after sperm penetration.** The objective of the present study was to determine the oxygen consumption and the REDOX status of zygotes and early embryos at the time of sperm penetration and cell cleavage and to investigate how metabolism relates to key temporal events and developmental competence. METHODS: Individual oxygen-consumption rates of bovine in vitro matured oocytes and presumptive zygotes (n = 101) were measured using the Nanorespirometer at 0, 7, 12, 17 and 24 h after IVF. RESULTS: **A peak of oxygen consumption was observed at the time of fertilization and a smaller rise and fall in oxygen consumption could be detected prior to the first cell cleavage. Increased reactive oxygen species (EMOD) production was also observed at 7 h and then at 24 h after IVF, just preceding the first embryonic cleavage. CONCLUSIONS: There are specific events during embryo development that appear to be associated with a change in oxygen consumption and REDOX state, indicating that both have a role in sperm-mediated oocyte activation and cell cleavage in bovine embryos.** (Lopes et al, 2010)

Sperm DNA fragmentation and oxidation are independent of malondialdehyde

There is clinical evidence to show that sperm DNA damage could be a marker of sperm quality and extensive data exist on the relationship between DNA damage and male fertility status. Detecting such damage in sperm could provide new elements besides semen parameters in diagnosing male infertility. We aimed to assess sperm DNA fragmentation and oxidation and to study the association between these two markers, routine semen parameters and malondialdehyde formation. METHODS: Semen samples from 55 men attending the Histology-Embryology Laboratory of Sfax Faculty of Medicine, Tunisia, for semen investigations were analyzed for sperm DNA fragmentation and oxidation using flow cytometry. The Sperm was also assessed spectrophotometrically for malondialdehyde formation. RESULTS: Within the studied group, 21 patients were nonasthenozoospermic (sperm motility $\geq$ 50%) and 34 patients were considered asthenozoospermic (sperm motility < 50%). A positive correlation was found between sperm DNA fragmentation and oxidation ($p = 0.01$; $r = 0.33$). We also found a negative correlation between sperm DNA fragmentation and some sperm parameters: total motility ($p = 0.001$; $r = -0.43$), rapid progressive motility (type a motility) ($p = 0.04$; $r = -0.27$), slow progressive motility (type b motility) ($p = 0.03$; $r = -0.28$), and vitality ($p < 0.001$; $r = -0.65$). Sperm DNA fragmentation was positively correlated with coiled tail ($p = 0.01$; $r = 0.34$). The two parameters that were found to be correlated with oxidative DNA damage were leucocytes concentrations ($p = 0.01$; $r = 0.38$) and broken neck ($p = 0.02$; $r = 0.29$). **Sperm MDA levels were** negatively correlated with sperm concentration ($p < 0.001$; $r = -0.57$), total motility ($p = 0.01$; $r = -0.35$) and type a motility ($p = 0.03$; $r = -0.32$); but **not correlated with DNA fragmentation and DNA oxidation. CONCLU-** SIONS: Our results support the evidence that **oxidative stress plays a key role in inducing DNA damage; but nuclear alterations and malondialdehyde don't seem to be synchronous.** (Zribi et al, 2011). **This study speaks volumes and refutes the reams of papers stating that EMODs are causative of sperm DNA damage.**

CHAPTER TWENTY THREE

Antioxidants in the food supply

Stacking of antioxidants

Check the ingredients of **margarine, dairy blends, crackers, biscuits, bread, baked goods, croissants, potato crisps, snack foods, muesli bars, crushed garlic in oil, soymilk and other processed foods** for likely antioxidant additives. But, they may not be labeled.

Harmful antioxidants (310-312) (319-321)

310 - Propyl gallate; 311 - Octyl gallate; 312 - Dodecyl gallate; 319 - tert-Butylhydroquinone, tBHQ; 320 - Butylated hydroxyanisole, BHA; 321 - Butylated hydroxytoluene, BHT.

Alternative antioxidants

300 - Ascorbic acid (vitamin C); 301 - Sodium ascorbate; 302 - Calcium ascorbate; 303 - Potassium ascorbate; 304 - Ascorbyl palmitate; 306 - Mixed tocopherols (vitamin E); 307 - dl-a-Tocopherol; 308 - g-Tocopherol; 309 - d-Tocopherol.

With restaurants in general or eating out, **any oils used to cook your food will almost certainly contain at least one of these potentially harmful antioxidant additives.**

Antioxidants that inhibit enzyme-catalyzed oxidation include agents that bind free oxygen (*i.e., reducing agents*), such as **ascorbic acid (vitamin C), and agents that inactivate the enzymes, such as citric acid and sulfites.**

Among antioxidants, the synthetic compounds **butylated hydroxyanisole (BHA), propyl gallate, ethoxyquin, and diphenylamine are commonly used as food additives.** Quercetin belongs to a large natural group of antioxidants, **the flavonoid family, with more than 6000 known members.**

Antioxidants added to food

Prior to the Civil War, people raised most of the food they ate and processing was limited to spices, salt and smoke. After the Civil War, the food supply system changed, cities grew, factories flourished and food manufacturers popped up. Scientific knowledge of food chemistry or antioxidants was practically nonexistent.

Antioxidants have diverse applications. They are used to prevent degradation in polymers, weakening in rubber and plastics, autoxidation and gum formation in gasoline, and discoloration of synthetic and natural pigments. They are used in foods, beverages, and cosmetic products to inhibit deterioration and spoilage.

Chemicals to keep products looking good until they were sold or to hide signs of spoilage were used without much restraint. Dangerous adulteration of foods became commonplace, such as the use of copper sulfate to keep vegetables appearance fresh and green and salicylic acid, borax and formaldehyde were also used dangerously.

Dr. Harvey Washington Wiley, chief chemist for the USDA was the predecessor to the FDA and he cautioned that the American people were being steadily poisoned by the dangerous chemicals that were being added to food with reckless abandon. In 1927 the Food, Drug and Insecticide Administration was created and later became the FDA.

It was not until 1958 that legislation was adopted requiring food and chemical manufactureresto test their additives before they were submitted to the FDA. Today, manufacturers are responsible for demonstrating their Generally Recognized as Safe (GRAS) status and providing evidence (such as scientific literature) to support it. Approximately 100 new substances are presented to the FDA for GRAS certification every year.

Food preservatives are classified into two main groups: antioxidants and anti-microbials.

Enzymes called phenolases catalyze the oxidation of certain molecules (*e.g.,* the amino acid tyrosine) when fruits and vegetables, such as apples, bananas, and potatoes, are cut or bruised. The product of these oxidation reactions, collectively known as enzymatic browning, is a dark pigment called melanin.

Commonly Used Chemical Preservatives Generally Recognized as Safe

Ascorbic acid
Ascorbyl palmitate
Benzoic acid
BHA
BHT
Calcium ascorbate
Calcium propionate
Calcium sorbate
Citrate acid
Dilauryl thiodipropionate
Distearyl thiodipropionate
Erythorbic acid
Ethoxyquin
Formic acid
Methylparaben
Potassium bisulphite
Potassium metabisulphite
Potassium sorbate
Propionic acid
Propul gallate
Propul paraben
Resin guaiae
Sodium ascorbate
Sodium benzoate
Sodium bisulphite
Sodium metabisulphite

Sodium nitrite
Sodium propionate
Sodium sorbate
Sodium sulphite
Sorbic acid
Stannous chloride
Sulphur dioxide
THBP - Trihydroxy-butyrophenone
TBHQ - Tertiary-butylhydroquinone
Thiodipinic acid
Tocopherols

Altogether too often, it is the practice to use levels of vitamin E far above the animals' nutrient requirement and the result is economically unfavorable. It has been shown in diets designed for chicken and turkey breeders that ethoxyquin has a vitamin E sparing effect.

Antioxidants prevent oxidative losses of vitamins A and E and pigmenters (oxy- and keto-cerotenoids) in stored mixed feeds. Antioxidants stabilize critical oxidation-susceptible nutrients that are naturally present in a fish feed composed of several feedstuffs so that losses are minimal from mixing and storing. If pig-menting substances are used, the anti-oxidants are definitely needed. The benefits of adequate, consistent use span all facets of fish production which include the processing and handling of feedstuffs, formulation, and fish cultural practices.

The U.S. Food and Drug Administration permits the following levels of anti-oxidant in finished feed:

(a) ethoxyquin (1,2 dihydro-6-ethoxy-2,2,4- trimethy quinoline): 150 ppm,
(b) BHT (butylated hydroxytoluene): 200 ppm, and
(c) BHA (butylated hydroxyanisole): 200 ppm.

A 2005 reassessment of inert ingredient tolerance of ethoxyquin was commis-sioned by the US Environmental Protection Agency (EPA). The reassessment states that "studies indicate that **ethoxyquin is toxic to aquatic invertebrates, and mildly toxic to fish" when ingested.**

Please realize that all of these antioxidants can contaminate animal products, such as eggs, milk, meat, etc. and the housing facilities or feed lots in which they are enclosed. Also, the antioxidant laced fish food is capable to contaminating the surrounding waters and ultimately getting into aquifers and municipal water supplies and create ecological disasters.

It is readily apparent that there are over 3 dozen antioxidants which may be added to feed stocks.

Flint River Ranch Pet Foods do not contain any of the following chemical preservatives, instead they use natural Vitamin E, a closely related fat-soluble compound known as Tocopherols. Their website states:

Ethoxyquin

- Promoted kidney carcinogenesis.

- Significantly increased incidence of stomach tumors.

- Enhanced bladder carcinogenesis.

BHA

- Enhanced stomach and urinary bladder carcinogenesis.

- Causes squamous-cell carcinomas in stomachs.

(Cancers of this type are among the most lethal and fastest acting, the swiftest effects being seen among animals with light colored fur.)

BHT

- Promoted urinary bladder carcinogenesis.

- Could be a promoter of thyroid carcinogenesis.

Studies have noted that BHA and other antioxidants, particularly propyl gallate and ethoxyquin, showed additional effects in inducing stomach hyperplasia and cytotoxicity.

BHA and BHT are used in human and pet foods to keep fats from going rancid. Both have been linked to cancer in laboratory animals; it's unknown whether they cause the same in people and dogs. There is evidence that certain people may have difficulty metabolizing BHA and BHT, resulting in health and behavior changes. Again, we don't know if the same is true for our dogs.

According to Dr. Wendell Belfield, DVM practicing veterinarian for some 26 years, both BHA and BHT are known to cause liver and kidney dysfunction and are banned in some European countries. He adds that ethoxyquin is suspected of causing cancer.

Ethoxyquin is listed and identified as a hazardous chemical by OSHA. It has a rating of 3 on a scale of 1 to 6, with 6 being super toxic requiring less than 7 drops to cause death. When manufactured by Monsanto, the containers are marked with the word POISON. **Monsanto makes no representations and will not be responsible for damages of any nature whatsoever.** The Department of Agriculture lists and controls Ethoxyquin as a pesticide.

In 1994, David A. Dzanis, D.V.M., Ph.D, said, "As Americans become more health conscious, they are reading food labels and choosing products more carefully. Many people are extending this scrutiny to food for their pets as well. Pet food labels are regulated by different rules than foods for human consumption, but reading and understanding a pet food label can help consumers make proper food choices for their pets, too.

According to a document produced by the Environmental Protection Agency (EPA), "Dogs are more susceptible to ethoxyquin toxicity than rats, with elevated liver enzymes and microscopic findings in the liver occurring at doses as low as 4 mg/kg/day over a 90-day feeding period."

The FDA and pet food industry officials defend the use of ethoxyquin, saying that ethoxyquin is safer than rancid fats. While this may be true, artificial preservatives are not the only way to prevent rancidity. In addition, if ethoxyquin is safe, why is it not permitted to be added to human foods (other than three spices), and why is the acceptable level for pet foods 50 times the residual amount allowed in human food?

How then can a consumer find out if their dog's food contains ethoxyquin, BHA, BHT, or other artificial preservatives? Unfortunately, there are no easy answers.

Commonly used feed antioxidants

Of the chemical compounds that have been investigated thus far, three have been found to be outstandingly effective antioxidants for feeds and feed ingredients and can be used both efficiently and economically. They are:

(a) Ethoxyquin (generic term: 1,2-dihydro-6-ethoxy-2,2,4- trimethylquinoline)
(b) BHA (butylated hydroxyanisole);
(c) BHT (butylated hydroxytoluene)

Ethoxyquin, however, has been demonstrated to be the most efficacious, followed closely by BHT and BHA.

With the advent of rations containing a high level of animal and vegetable fats, the requirement for antioxidant protection has become very apparent. The majority of studies over the last few years has focused on ethoxyquin as a preservative or antioxidant. **Other chemical preservatives are: ascorbic acid, propionic acid, benzoic acid, citric acid and their various salts.** There are technological problems (i.e., moisture level, etc.) associated with the use of these preservatives. Economics, however, remain the most important consideration which limit their use in fish foods.

Food (feed) antioxidants for animals and fish

Antioxidants prevent fat oxidation (rancidity). Rancidity creates off-flavors and off-odors which dramatically decrease palatability and food consumption. Antioxidants also prevent the destruction of several nutrients. They provide direct protection to a number of vitamins which are unstable to the effects of oxygen.

Natural antioxidants such as ascorbic acid (vitamin C) and vitamin E or other related tocopherols are effective antioxidants but are relatively short lived when compared to the chemical antioxidants. Due to the realities of the pet food distribution system and the relatively low volumes and slow use of exotic bird foods, the time interval between manufacturing a product and feeding it may be beyond the effective life of a natural antioxidant. If the product could be produced, refrigerated and consumed within a few months, natural antioxidants might be practical. But, since this time frame cannot be guaranteed, it seems prudent to manufacturers to use the more stable petro-chemical antioxidants for this critical function.

The commonly used chemical antioxidants, butylated hydroxyanisol (BHA), butylated hydroxytoluene (BHT) and ethoxyquin, are all chemicals that research indicates could be potential carcinogens when fed to certain species at high levels. The use of antioxidants has been questioned by scientists, pet owners and retailers.

Phenytoin induced oxidative stress in pre- and postnatal rat development - effect of vitamin E on selective biochemical variables (Navaroa et al, 2005)

A pre- and postnatal study was carried out to investigate the effect of high dose (500 mg/kg) of the natural antioxidant vitamin E (VIT E) on biochemical variables in the model of chronic intrauterine hypoxia. Chronic hypoxia was induced by administration of the anticonvulsant phenytoin (PHT) during pregnancy. Rats were orally treated with PHT (150 mg/kg) from day 7 to 18 of gestation and VIT E prior to PHT orally on the same days. The activity of the lysosomal enzyme N-acetyl-ss-D-glucosaminidase (NAGA) and the level of glutathione (GSH) were used as markers of tissue damage. In the prenatal study PHT-induced embryofoetal toxicity was associated with an increase in NAGA activity and decrease of GSH level in maternal serum and heart and with an increase in NAGA activity in the placenta. Administration of VIT E did not inhibit the above given changes. PHT increased the activity of NAGA and decreased the level of GSH in foetal organs (liver, lungs, brain). VIT E did not reverse these changes. In the postnatal study, we did not find any significant differences in NAGA activity in the organs of 1-day-old pups. An increase of liver GSH level was found in PHT and VIT E+PHT groups of pups and in the group VIT E+PHT in the lungs. In conclusion, **supplementation with a high-dose of VIT E failed to protect maternal, foetal and new-born rat organs from PHT induced changes of selective biochemical variables.** (Navaroa et al, 2005)

Synergistic carcinogenic effect of antioxidants

Once again, we see the harmful potential of common antioxidants. Cumulatively, they may combine to produce an overall weakened state with an EMOD insuffiency, which allows for the manifestation of a wide range of disease conditions.

The carcinogenicity of low dietary levels of the antioxidants butylated hydroxyanisole (BHA), caffeic acid, sesamol, 4-methoxyphenol (4-MP) and catechol, known to target the forestomach or glandular stomach, were examined alone or in combination in a 2-year long-term experiment and their modifying effects assessed in a medium-term multiorgan rat model. In the carcinogenicity study, slightly increased incidences of fore-stomach papillomas were found in the sesamol- (15.8%), caffeic acid- (14.8%), catechol- (3%) and 4-MP- (11.5%)

treated groups as compared with basal diet (0%), and **a significant increase was observed with the five antioxidants in combination** (42.9%, P < 0.001). In the low dose case, the incidence of fore-stomach papillomas was significantly increased only in the combination group. The results indicate that **even at low dose levels phenolic compounds can exert additive/synergistic effect on carcinogenesis** (Hirose et al, 1998).

The synthetic antioxidant BHA was first found to exert carcinogenic potential in rat and hamster fore-stomach epithelium. Many antioxidants have been shown to modify carcinogenesis, and as a rule, they inhibit the initiation stage by reducing the interaction between carcinogen and DNA. However, both promotion and inhibition have been reported for second-stage carcinogenesis, depending on the organ site, species of animal, or initiating carcinogen (Ito and Hirose, 1989).

The anti-oxidant food additive, butylated hydroxytoluene (BHT) was fed to rats and BHT resulted in a significant increase in liver weight. The liver cells presented gradual vacuolization, cytoplasmic disintegration, "moth-eaten" appearance, ballooning degeneration, hepatocellular necrosis, aggregation of chromatin material around the periphery of the nuclear envelope, SER prolif- eration, RER clumping with broken cisternae, withered and autolyzed mito- chondria, augmentation of lipid droplets and glycogen depletion (Safer and ak-Nughamish, 1999).

And lastly, since there is widespread use of antioxidants in the food process- ing industries, especially oil and oil based ones and since the ban on the fur- ther usage of butylated hydroxyanisole (BHA) and butylated hydroxytoluene (BHT) by the Food and Agriculture Organization of the United Nations (FAO) in 1980, there have been several reports indicating that BHA and BHT might have detrimental effects. BHT is more toxic than BHA and this rat study clearly indicates that at the concentrations of 0.75%, BHA and BHT are harmful to the blood (Jayalakshmi and Sharma, 1986).

Genistein and isoflavone risks

There are concern of *genotoxicity associated with higher levels of genistein exposure* that are typically not achievable through dietary intake, with most of these data obtained from *in vitro* experiments using cells in culture. For example, *genistein exposure of L5178Y mouse lymphoma cells at concentrations less than 100 nM induced micronuclei formation and mutagenesis at the thymidine kinase locus.* (Boos, Stopper, 2000) *and chronic exposure (3 months) of human MCF-10A cells induced genomic instability.* (Kim et al, 2008)

It has also been found that *genistein at higher concentrations could also result in DNA damage detectable by either the comet assay or the chromosomal aberrations in both cells in culture* (Pool-Zobel et al, 2000) (Michael et al, 2006) *and in human sperm and lymphocytes obtained from donors.* (Anderson et al, 1997) (Kulling et al, 1999)

These genotoxic effects have been attributed, at least in part, to the known role of genistein in inhibiting topoisomerase II. (Markovits et al, 1989)

Genistein may have *possible harmful effects on reproductive health. A wide range of reproductive biological and behavioral defects were observed in male rats fed a genistein supplemented diet* (Wisniewski et al, 2003) and *recent data have demonstrated a direct effect of genistein on Leydig cells.* (Hancock et al, 2009) (Sherrill et al, 2010)

Providing physiologically relevant doses of genistein (i.e. those achievable through dietary intake) neonatally resulted in a wide range of defects in the developing female reproductive system and this has been extensively reviewed by Jefferson et al.. (Jefferson et al, 2006)

Additional concerns about possible teratogenic effects of genistein have been raised in the studies using zebrafish. (Kim et al, 2009) (Sassi-Messai et al, 2009)

There is a serious concern as to whether genistein supplementation can have an adverse effect on cancer survival. An extensive and comprehensive review of the preclinical and clinical literature on both the benefits and the possible risks of genistein has been published by Tayor et al. (Taylor, Levy et al, 2009)

Although several reports have indicated that genistein could stimulate the growth of the ER^+ human breast cancer cell line MCF-7, *it was shown early on that genistein concentrations as low as 10–100 nM can be growth stimulatory* with higher concentrations of $20 \mu M$ being inhibitory, presumably due to toxicity. (Hsieh et al, 19980

In that regard, *genistein supplementation enhanced mammary gland growth and tumor development of estrogen-dependent MCF7 cells in athymic mice in a dose-dependent manner* (Allred et al, 2001) *and when ovariectomized mice were treated with the chemical carcinogen 1-methyl-1-nitrosourea to induce mammary tumorigenesis.* (Allred et al, 2004)

Supplementation studies conducted in humans have raised the possibility that soy may promote breast cancer development.

In a trial that randomized women with benign or malignant breast disease to soy supplementation (60 g of soy containing 45 mg of isoflavones) or their normal diet daily for 2 wk, women receiving the soy supplements had increased serum genistein levels in comparison to women on a standard diet, and their histologically normal breast tissue exhibited enhanced breast epithelial cell proliferation and significantly increased progesterone receptor levels. (McMichael-Phillips et al, 1998)

In general, **the data suggest that short-term exposure to soy caused a weak estrogenic effect.**

An additional concern about the potential harm that might be done by genistein stems from data that it can stimulate proliferation of tamoxifen-sensitive cells (Ju et al, 2008)

(Ju et al, 2002) (Limer et al, 2006) *and attenuate the anti-tumor activities of both tamoxifen* (Liu et al, 2005) *and the aromatase inhibitor letrozole in mouse models of breast cancer.* (Ju et al, 2008)

Consequently, *there remains some concern regarding genistein's possible genotoxic, teratogenic, and proestrogenic activity at high concentrations, and therefore its long-term safety as a dietary supplement.*

Genistein may have very different effects on healthy breast tissue as compared with breast cancers, and this may be further complicated by the ER status of the tumor. There is also a possibility of an interaction between genistein and common approaches to manage breast cancer (tamoxifen and letrozole) that reduce the efficacy of these drugs. In addition, it is important to consider attainable physiological doses of genistein in humans when assessing its safety. Serum levels of genistein from soy consumption or supplementation are typically below $5\,\mu M$, with many of the reports of growth stimulation of cells in culture involving concentrations ranging from 0.01 to $10\,\mu M$ and the growth inhibitory and genotoxic effects occur at higher concentrations.

References

(Aasebo et al, 1993) (Aasebo U, et al. Reversal of sexual impotence in male patients with chronic obstructive pulmonary disease and hypoxemia with long-term oxygen therapy. J Steroid Biochem Mol Biol. 1993 Dec;46(6):799-803)

(Adler et al., 1999) (Adler V, Yin Z, Tew KD, Ronai Z. Role of redox potential and reactive oxygen species in stress signaling. *Oncogene.* 1999;18:6104–6111)

(Adamopoulos et al, 2006) (Adamopoulos D, Venaki E, Koukkou E, et al. Association of carotene rich diet with hypogonadism in a male athlete. *Asian J Androl.* 2006;8:488–492)

(Adeniyi et al, 2007) (Adeniyi AA, Brindley GS, Pryor JP, Ralph DJ. Yohimbine in the treatment of orgasmic dysfunction. Asian J Andol. 2007 May;9(3):403-7)

(Agarwal, Said, 2004) (Agarwal A, Said TM. Carnitines and male infertility. *Reprod Biomed Online.* 2004; 8: 376 -384)

(Agarwal, Saleh, 2002) (Agarwal A, Saleh RA. Role of oxidants in male infertility: rationale, significance, and treatment. *Urol Clin North Am.* 2002;29: 817 -827)

(Agarwal et al, 2003) (Agarwal A, Saleh RA, Bedaiwy MA. Role of reactive oxygen species in the pathophysiology of human reproduction. *Fertility and Sterility.* 2003;79(4):829–843)

(Agarwal et al, 2004) (Agarwal A, Nallella KP, Allamaneni SSR, Said TM. Role of antioxidants in treatment of male infertility: an overview of the literature. *Reproductive BioMedicine Online.* 2004;8(6):616–627)

(Agarwal et al, 2005) (Agarwal A, Prabakaran SA, and Said TM. Prevention of oxidative stress injury to sperm. Journal of Andrology, Vol. 26, No. 6, November/December 2005)

(Agarwal, Gupta, et al, 2005) (Agarwal A, Gupta S, Sharma RK. Role of oxidative stress in female reproduction. *Reproductive Biology and Endocrinology.* 2005;3, article 28)

(Agarwal, Prabakaran, 2005) (Agarwal A, Prabakaran SA. Mechanism, measurement, and prevention of oxidative stress in male reproductive physiology. *Indian Journal of Experimental Biology.* 2005;43(11):963–974)

(Agarwal et al, 2008) (Agarwal A, Makker K, Sharma R. Clinical relevance of oxidative stress in male factor infertility: an update. *American Journal of Reproductive Immunology.* 2008;59(1):2–11)

(Aitken, Clarkson, 1988) (Aitken RJ, Clarkson JS. Significance of reactive oxygen species and antioxidants in defining the efficacy of sperm preparation techniques. *J Androl.* 1988;9: 367 -376)

(Aitken et al, 1992) (Aitken RJ, Buckingham D, West K, Wu FC, Zikopoulos K, Richardson DW. Differential contribution of leucocytes and spermatozoa to the generation of reactive oxygen species in the ejaculates of oligozoospermic patients and fertile donors. *J Reprod Fertil.* 1992; 94: 451 -462)

(Aitken, 1997) (Aitken RJ. Molecular mechanisms regulating human sperm function. *Molecular Human Reproduction.* 1997;3(3):169–173)

(Aitken, Fisher, et al, 1997) (Aitken RJ, Fisher HM, Fulton N, et al. Reactive oxygen species generation by human spermatozoa is induced by exogenous NADPH and inhibited by the flavoprotein inhibitors diphenylene iodonium and quinacrine. *Molecular Reproduction and Development.* 1997;47(4):468–482)

(Aitken, Fisher, 1994) (Aitken J, Fisher H. Reactive oxygen species generation and human spermatozoa: the balance of benefit and risk. Bioessays. 1994;16:259–67)

(Aitken et al, 2004) (Aitken RJ, Ryan AL, Baker MA, McLaughlin EA. Redox activity associated with the maturation and capacitation of mammalian spermatozoa. *Free Radic Biol Med.* 2004; 36: 994 -1010)

(Aitken et al, 1995) (Aitken RJ, Baker HWG. Seminal leukocytes: passengers, terrorists or good Samaritans ? *Human Reproduction.* 1995;10(7):1736–1739)

(Aitken, Roman, 2008) (R John Aitken and Shaun D Roman. Antioxidant systems and oxidative stress in the testes. Oxid Med Cell Longev. 2008 Oct-Dec; 1(1): 15–24)

(Aitken et al, 2009) (Aitken RJ, De Iuliis GN, McLachlan RI. Biological and clinical significance of DNA damage in the male germ line. Int J Androl. 2009;32:46–56)

(Aitken, De Luliis, 2010) (Aitken R.J. and De Luliis GN. On the possible origins of DNA damage in human spermatozoa. Mol Hum. Reprod. (2010) Vol. 16, Issue 1, Pp. 3-13)

(Alaily, 2000) (Alaily A. Obstetrics and gynaecology in ancient and modern Egypt. Rosewell Publishing, 2000)

(Allamaneni et al, 2004) (Allamaneni SS, Naughton CK, Sharma RK, Thomas AJ Jr, Agarwal A. Increased seminal reactive oxygen species levels in patients with varicoceles correlate with varicocele grade but not with testis size. *Fertil Steril.* 2004;82: 1684 -1686)

(Alleva et al, 1997) (Alleva R, Scararmucci A, Mantero F, Bompadre S, Leoni L, Littarru GP. The protective role of ubiquinol-10 against formation of lipid hydroperoxides in human seminal fluid. *Mol Aspects Med.* 1997;18(suppl): S221 -S228)

(Allred et al, 2001) (Allred, C. D., Allred, K. F., Ju, Y. H., Virant, S. M., Helferich, W. G., Soy diets containing varying amounts of genistein stimulate growth of estrogen-dependent (MCF-7) tumors in a dose-dependent manner. Cancer Res. 2001, 61, 5045–5050)

(Allred et al, 2004) (Allred, C. D., Allred, K. F., Ju, Y. H., Clausen, L. M. et al., Dietary genistein results in larger MNU-induced, estrogen-dependent mammary tumors following ovariectomy of Sprague-Dawley rats. Carcinogenesis 2004, 25, 211–218)

(Alverez et al, 1987) (Alvarez JG, Touchstone JC, Blasco L, Storey BT. Spontaneous lipid peroxidation and production of hydrogen peroxide and superoxide in human spermatozoa. Superoxide dismutase as major enzyme protectant against oxygen toxicity. J Androl. 1987;8:338–48)

(Angulo et al, 2010)(Angulo J, Wright HM, Cuevas P. Nebivolol Dilates Human Penile Arteries and Reverses Erectile Dysfunction in Diabetic Rats through Enhancement of Nitric Oxide Signaling. J Sex Med. 2010 Aug;7(8):2681-97)

(Anderson et al, 1997) (Anderson, D., Dobrzynska, M. M., Basaran, N., Effect of various genotoxins and reproductive toxins in human lymphocytes and sperm in the Comet assay. Teratog. Carcinog. Mutagen. 1997, 17, 29–43)

(Anderson et al, 2003) (Anderson D, Schmid TE, Baumgartner A, Cemeli-Carratala E, Brinkworth MH, Wood JM. Oestrogenic compounds and oxidative stress (in human sperm and lymphocytes in the Comet assay). Mutat Res. 2003;544:173–8)

(Andersson, 2003)(Andersson KE. Erectile physiological and pathophysiological pathways involved in erectile dysfunction. J Urol. Aug 2003;170(2 Pt 2):S6-13; discussion S13-4)

(Appasamy et al, 2007) (Appasamy M, Muttukrishna S, Pizzey AR, Ozturk O, Groome NP, Serhal P, et al. Relationship between male reproductive hormones, sperm DNA damage and markers of oxidative stress in infertility. Reprod Biomed Online. 2007;14:159–65)

(Aslan et al., 2003) (Aslan M, Ozben T. Oxidants in receptor tyrosine kinase signal transduction pathways. Antioxid Redox Signal. 2003;5:781–788)

(Attaran et al, 2000) (Attaran M, Pasqualotto E, Falcone T, et al. The effect of follicular fluid reactive oxygen species on the outcome of in vitro fertilization. International Journal of Fertility and Women's Medicine. 2000;45(5):314–320)

(Audet et al, 2004) (Audet I, LaForest JP, Martineau GP, Matte JJ. Effect of vitamin supplements on some aspects of performance, vitamin status, and semen quality in boars. 2004. J. Anim. Sci. 82(2):626-33)

(Aufderheide, 2003) (Aufderheide AC. The scientific study of mummies. Cambridge University Press, 2003)

(Awda et al, 2009) (Awda BJ, et al, Reactive oxygen species and boar sperm function. Biol Reprod. 2009 Sep;81(3):553-61)

(Babior et al., 1999) (Babior BM. NADPH oxidase: an update. *Blood.* 1999;93:1464–1476)

(Baker et al, 2011) (Baker LH et al. Vitamin E and the risk of prostate cancer: the Selenium and Vitamin E Cancer Prevention Trial (SELECT). *JAMA.* 2011;306:1549-1556)

(Bagi et al, 2003) (Bagi Z, Koller A, Kaley G. Superoxide-NO interaction decreases flow- and agonist-induced dilations of coronary arterioles in Type 2 diabetes mellitus. *Am J Physiol Heart Circ Physiol* 285: H1404–H1410, 2003)

(Bankson et al, 1993) (Bankson DD, Kestin M, Rifai N. Role of free radicals in cancer and atherosclerosis. *Clin Lab Med.* 1993; 13: 463 -480)

(Bansal, Bilaspuri, 2007) (Bansal AK, Bilaspuri GS. Effect of ferrous ascorbate on *in vitro* capacitation and acrosome reaction in cattle bull spermatozoa. *Animal Science Report.* 2007;1(2):69–77)

(Bansal, Bilaspuri, 2010) (Bansal AK, Bilaspuri GS. Impacts of oxidative stress and antioxidants on semen functions. Vet Med Int. 2010 Sep 7;2010. pii: 686137)

(Barroso et al, 2000) (Barroso G, Morshedi M, Oehninger S. Analysis of DNA fragmentation, plasma membrane translocation of phosphatidylserine and oxidative stress in human spermatozoa. Hum Reprod. 2000;15:1338–44)

(Behr-Roussel, 2004) (Behr-Roussel D. Cardiovascular risk factors, erection disorders and endothelium dysfunction. J Soc Biol. 2004;198(3):237-41)

(Bilodeau et al, 2000) (Bilodeau JF, Chatterjee S, Sirard MA, Gagnon C. Levels of antioxidant defenses are decreased in bovine spermatozoa after a cycle of freezing and thawing. *Mol Reprod Dev.* 2000; 55: 282 -288)

(Biswas, Deb, 1965) (Biswas NM, Deb C. Testicular degeneration in rats during hypervitaminosis A. *Endokrinologie.* 1965;49:64–69)

(Boos, Stopper, 2000) (Boos, G., Stopper, H., Genotoxicity of several clinically used topoisomerase II inhibitors. Toxicol. Lett. 2000, 116, 7–16)

(Bucak et al, 2007) (Bucak MN, Ateşşahin A, Varişli O, Yüce A, Tekin N, Akçay A. The influence of trehalose, taurine, cysteamine and hyaluronan on ram semen. Microscopic and oxidative stress parameters after freeze-thawing process. *Theriogenology.* 2007;67(5):1060–1067)

(Bucak et al, 2008) (Bucak MN, Ateşşahin A, Yüce A. Effect of anti-oxidants and oxidative stress parameters on ram semen after the freeze-thawing process. *Small Ruminant Research.* 2008;75(2-3):128–134)

(Bucak et al, 2010) (Bucak MN, Sariözkan S, Tuncer PB, et al. The effect of antioxidants on post-thawed Angora goat (Capra hircus ancryrensis) sperm parameters, lipid peroxidation and antioxidant activities. *Small Ruminant Research.* 2010;89(1):24–30)

(Carrell, Liu, 2001) (Carrell DT, Liu L. Altered protamine 2 expression is uncommon in donors of known fertility, but common among men with poor fertilizing capacity, and may reflect other abnormalities of spermiogenesis. J Androl. 2001;22:604–10)

(Cemeli et al, 2004) (Cemeli E, Schmid TE, Anderson D. Modulation by flavonoids of DNA damage induced by estrogen-like compounds. Environ Mol Mutagen. 2004;44:420–6)

(Chatterjee, Gagnon, 2001) (Chatterjee S, Gagnon C. Production of reactive oxygen species by spermatozoa undergoing cooling, freezing, and thawing. *Molecular Reproduction and Development.* 2001;59(4):451–458)

(Chen et al, 1999) (Chen J, Wollman Y, Chernichovsky T, Iaina A, Sofer M, Matzkin H. Effect of oral administration of high-dose nitric oxide donor L-arginine in men with organic erectile dysfunction: results of a double-blind, randomized, placebo-controlled study. *BJU Int.* Feb 1999;83(3):269-73)

(Chi et al, 2008) (Chi HJ, Kim JH, Ryu CS, Lee JY, Park JS, Chung DY, et al. Protective effect of antioxidant supplementation in sperm-preparation medium against oxidative stress in human spermatozoa. Hum Reprod. 2008;23:1023–8)

(Chitaley et al, 2001) (Chitaley K, Webb RC, Mills TM. RhoA/Rho-kinase: a novel player in the regulation of penile erection. *Int J Impot Res.* Apr 2001;13(2):67-72)

(Dandona et al, 2001) (Paresh Dandona et al. Acute suppressive effect of hydrocortisone on p47[phox] subunit of nicotinamide adenine dinucleotide phosphate oxidase. Metabolism. Volume 50, Issue 5, May 2001, Pages 548-552)

(Darley-Usmar et al, 1995) (Darley-Usmar V, Wiseman H, Halliwell B. Nitric oxide and oxygen radicals: a question of balance. *FEBS Letters.* 1995;369(2-3):131–135)

(Davies et al., 1999) (Davies KJ. The broad spectrum of responses to oxidants in proliferating cells: A new paradigm for oxidative stress. *IUBMB Life.* 1999;48:41–47)

(Davies, 2000) (Davies KJ. Oxidative stress, antioxidant defenses, and damage removal, repair, and replacement systems. *IUBMB Life.* 2000; 50: 279 -289)

(Dawson et al, 1987) (Dawson EB, Harris WA, Rankin WE, Charpentier LA, McGanity WJ. Effect of ascorbic acid on male fertility. *Ann N Y Acad Sci.* 1987;498: 312 -323)

(de Lamirande, Gagnon, 1993) (de Lamirande E, Gagnon C. A positive role for the superoxide anion in triggering hyperactivation and capacitation of human spermatozoa. *International Journal of Andrology.* 1993;16(1):21–25)

(de Lamirande, Gagnon, 1993) (de Lamirande E, Gagnon C. A positive role for the superoxide anion in triggering hyperactivation and capacitation of human spermatozoa. *International Journal of Andrology.* 1993;16(1):21–25)

(de Lamirande, Gagnon, 1995) (de Lamirande E, Gagnon C. Impact of reactive oxygen species on spermatozoa: a balancing act between beneficial and detrimental effects. *Human Reproduction.* 1995;10(supplement 1):15–21)

(de Lamirande et al, 1997) (de Lamirande E, Leclerc P, Gagnon C. Capacitation as a regulatory event that primes spermatozoa for the acrosome reaction and fertilization. *Molecular Human Reproduction.* 1997;3(3):175–194)

(de Lamirande et al, 1998) (de Lamirande E, Tsai C, Harakat A, Gagnon C. Involvement of reactive oxygen species in human sperm arcosome reaction induced by A23187, lysophosphatidylcholine, and biological fluid ultrafiltrates. *J Androl.* 1998;19: 585 -594)

(Delbes et al, 2010) (Delbes G et al, Toxicants and human sperm chromatin integrity. Mol. Hum. reprod. (2010)16(1):14-22)

(Depuydt et al, 1998) (Depuydt C, Zalata A, Christophe A, Mahmoud A, Comhaire F. Mechanisms of sperm deficiency in male accessory gland infection. *Andrologia.* 1998; 30(suppl 1): 29 -33)

(Desai et al, 2009) (Desai N, Sharma R, Maker K, Sabnegh E, Agarwal A. Physiological and pathological levels of reactive oxygen species in neat semen of infertile men. *Fertility and Sterility.* 2009;92:1626–1631)

(de Yebra et al, 1993) (de Yebra L, Ballesca JL, Vanrell JA, Bassas L, Oliva R. Complete selective absence of protamine P2 in humans. J Biol Chem. 1993;268:10553–7)

(Di Mascio et al, 1989) (Di Mascio P, Kaiser S, Sies H. Lycopene as the most efficient biological carotenoid singlet oxygen quencher. *Arch Biochem Biophys.* 1989;274: 532 -538)

(Dobrzynska et al, 2004) (Dobrzynska MM, Baumgartner A, Anderson D. Antioxidants modulate thyroid hormone- and noradrenaline-induced DNA damage in human sperm. Mutagenesis. 2004;19:325–30)

(Donnelley et al, 1999) (Donnelly ET, McClure N, Lewis SE. The effect of ascorbate and alpha-tocopherol supplementation in vitro on DNA integrity and hydrogen peroxide-induced DNA damage in human spermatozoa. Mutagenesis. 1999;14:505–12)

(Donnelly et al, 2000) (Donnelly ET, et al. Glutathione and hypotaurine in vitro: effects on human sperm motility, DNA integrity and production of reactive oxygen species. Mutagenesis. 2000 Jan;15(1):61-8)

(du Plessis et al, 2008) (du Plessis SS, Makker K, Desai NR, Agarwal A. Impact of oxidative stress on IVF. *Expert Review of Obstetrics and Gynecology.* 2008;3(4):539–554)

(Erdei et al, 2006) (Erdei N, Tóth A, Pásztor ET, Papp Z, Edes I, Koller A, Bagi Z. High-fat diet-induced reduction in nitric oxide-dependent arteriolar dilation in rats: role of xanthine oxidase-derived superoxide anion. *Am J Physiol Heart Circ Physiol* 291: H2107–H2115, 2006)

(Estes, 1993) (Estes JW. The medical skills of ancient Egypt. Science History Publications, 1993)

(Finkel, 2011) (Finkel T. Signal transduction by reactive oxygen species. JCB Home. 2011 Archive. 11 July. 194(1): 7)

(Ford, 2001) (Ford WC. Reactive oxygen species and sperm. *Human Fertility.* 2001;4:77–78)

(Ford, Whittington, 1998) (Ford WC, Whittington K. Antioxidant treatment for male subfertility: a promise that remains unfulfilled. *Hum Reprod.* 1998;13: 1416 -1419)

(Fraga et al, 1991) (Fraga CG, Motchnik PA, Shigenaga MK, Helbock HJ, Jacob RA, Ames BN. Ascorbic acid protects against endogenous oxidative DNA damage in human sperm. Proc Natl Acad Sci U S A. 1991;88:11003–6)

(Gabriele et al, 2006) (Gabriele Fröböse, Rolf Fröböse, Michael Gross (Translator): *Lust and Love: Is it more than Chemistry?* Publisher: Royal Society of Chemistry, ISBN 0-85404-867-7, 2006)

(Gagnon et al, 1991) (Gagnon C, Iwasaki A, De Lamirande E, Kovalski N. Reactive oxygen species and human spermatozoa. *Annals of the New York Academy of Sciences.* 1991;637:436–444)

(Gao et al, 2009) (Gao Q, Zhao X, Ahmad M, Wolin MS. Mitochondrial-derived hydrogen peroxide inhibits relaxation of bovine coronary arterial smooth muscle to hypoxia through stimulation of ERK MAP kinase. *Am J Physiol Heart Circ Physiol* 297: H2262–H2269, 2009)

(Garrido et al, 2004) (Garrido N, Meseguer M, Simon C, et al. Prooxidative and antioxidative imbalance in human semen and its relation with male infertility. *Asian Journal of Andrology.* 2004;6(1):59–65)

(Genova et al., 2004) (Genova ML, Pich MM, Bernacchia A, Bianchi C, Biondi A, Bovina C, Falasca AI, Formiggini G, Castelli GP, Lenaz G. The mitochondrial production of reactive oxygen species in relation to aging and pathology. *Ann NY Acad Sci.* 2004;1011:86–100)

(Ghalioungui et al, 1963) (Ghalioungui P, Khalil SH, Ammar AR. On an ancient Egyptian method of diagnosing pregnancy and determining foetal sex. Med Hist 1963;7:241-6)

(Gharagozloo, Aitken, 2011) (Gharagozloo P, Aitken RJ. The role of sperm oxidative stress in male infertility and the significance of oral antioxidant therapy. Hum Reprod. 2011 Jul;26(7):1628-40)

(Gil-Villa et al, 2008) (Gil-Villa AM, Cardona-Maya W, Agarwal A, Sharma R, Cadavid A. Role of male factor in early recurrent embryo loss: do antioxidants have any effect? Fertil Steril 2008)

(Gleichert et al, 1971) (Gleichert JE. Etienne Joseph Jacquemin, discoverer of "Chadwick's sign". J Hist Med Allied Sci 1971;26:75-80)

(Gomez et al, 1996) (Gomez E, Buckingham DW, Brindle J, Lanzafame F, Irvine DS, Aitken RJ. Development of an image analysis system to monitor the retention of residual cytoplasm by human spermatozoa: correlation with biochemical markers of the cytoplasmic space, oxidative stress, and sperm function. *J Androl.* 1996;17: 276 -287)

(Goncalves et al, 2010) (Gonçalves F, Barretto LSS, Arruda RP, Perri SHV, Mingoti GZ. Effect of antioxidants during bovine *in vitro* fertilization procedures on spermatozoa and embryo development. *Reproduction in Domestic Animals.* 2010;45(1):129–135)

(Greco, Iacobelli, et al, 2005) (Greco E, Iacobelli M, Rienzi L, Ubaldi F, Ferrero S, Tesarik J. Reduction of the incidence of sperm DNA fragmentation by oral antioxidant treatment. J Androl. 2005;26:349–53)

(Greco, Romano et al, 2005) (Greco E, Romano S, Iacobelli M, Ferrero S, Baroni E, Minasi MG, et al. ICSI in cases of sperm DNA damage: beneficial effect of oral antioxidant treatment. Hum Reprod. 2005;20:2590–4)

(Griendling et al., 1999) (Griendling KK, Harrison DG. Dual role of reactive oxygen species in vascular growth. *Circ Res.* 1999;85:562–563)

(Guerin et al, 2001) (Guérin P, El Mouatassim S, Ménézo Y. Oxidative stress and protection against reactive oxygen species in the pre-implantation embryo and its surroundings. *Human Reproduction Update.* 2001;7(2):175–189)

(Gupta et al, 2007) (Gupta S, Agarwal A, Banerjee J. et al. The role of oxidative stress in spontaneous abortion and recurrent pregnancy loss: a systematic review. Obstet Gynecol Surv. 2007 May;62(5):335-47; quiz 353-4)

(Guzik et al, 2002) (Guzik TJ, West NE, Pillai R, Taggart DP, Channon KM. Nitric oxide modulates superoxide release and peroxynitrite formation in human blood vessels. *Hypertension* 39: 1088–1094, 2002)

(Guzik et al, 2004) (Guzik TJ, Sadowski J, Kapelak B, Jopek A, Rudzinski P, Pillai R, Korbut R, Channon KM. Systemic regulation of vascular NAD(P) H oxidase activity and nox isoform expression in human arteries and veins. *Arterioscler Thromb Vasc Biol* 24: 1614–1620, 2004)

(Haddad et al., 2002) (Haddad JJ. Antioxidant and prooxidant mechanisms in the regulation of redox(y)-sensitive transcription factors. *Cell Signal.* 2002;14:879–897)

(Haimov-Kochman et al, 2005) (Haimov-Kochman R, Sciaky-Tamir Y, Hurwitz A. Reproduction concepts and practices in ancient Egypt mirrored by modern medicine. Eur J Ostet Gynaecol Reprod Biol 2005;123:3-8)

(Hancock et al, 2009) (Hancock, K. D., Coleman, E. S., Tao, Y. X., Morrison, E. E. et al., Genistein decreases androgen biosynthesis in rat Leydig cells by interference with luteinizing hormone-dependent signaling. Toxicol. Lett. 2009, 184, 169–175)

(Hampl et al, 2004) (Hampl JS, Taylor CA, Johnston CS. Vitamin C deficiency and depletion in the United States: the Third National Health and Nutrition Examination Survey, 1988 to 1994. Am J Public Health. 2004;94:870–5)

(Hao and Maret, 2005) (Hao Q, Maret W. Imbalance between pro-oxidant and pro-antioxidant functions of zinc in disease. J Alzheimers Dis. 2005 Nov;8(2):161-70; discussion 209-15)

(Harayama et al, 1998) (Harayama H, Miyake M, Shidara O, Iwamoto E, Kato S. Effects of calcium and bicarbonate on head-to-head agglutination in ejaculated boar spermatozoa. Reprod Fert Dev 1998;10:445-50)

(Harman, 1956) (Harman D. Aging: a theory based on free radical and radiation chemistry. J Gerontol 11: 298–300, 1956).

(Harman, 1957) (Harman, D. 1957. Prolongation of the normal life span by radiation protection chemicals. J. Gerontol. 12: 257-263)

(Harman, Lancet, 1961) (Harman D. 1961. Mutation, cancer and aging. Lancet I: 200-201).

(Harman, cancer, 1961) (Harman, D. 1961. Prolongation of the normal life span and inhibition of spontaneous cancer by antioxidants. J. Gerontol. 16: 147-154)

(Harman, 1968) (Harman D. Free radical theory of aging: effect of free radical reaction inhibitors on the mortality rate of male LAF mice. *J Gerontol A Biol Sci Med Sci* 23: 476-482, 1968).

(Harman, 1972) (Harman, D. (1972) "The biological clock: the mitochondria?" J Am Geriatr Soc 20: 145-47).

(Harman, 1981) (Harman D., 1981. The aging process. Proc. Natl Acad. Sci. USA 78, 7124–7128).

(Harman, 1984) (Harman D. Free radical theory of aging: the free radical diseases. Age 7: 111-131, 1984).

(Harman, 1987) (Harman, D. H.. Free radical theory of aging: effects of antioxidants on mitochondrial function. *Age* 10: 58-61, 1987).

(Harman, *In* Lipofuscin. 1988) (Harman, D. 1988. Free radical theory of aging, current status. *In* Lipofuscin - 1987, State of the Art. I. Zs.-Nagy, Ed.:3-21. Akadémiai Kiadò, Budapest; Elsevier Science Publishers, Amsterdam)

(Harman, 1992) (Harman, D. 1992. Role of free radicals in aging and disease. Ann. N.Y. Acad. Sci. 673: 126-141)

(Harman, 1994) (Harman, D. 1994. Free radical theory of aging. Increasing the functional life span. Ann. N.Y. Acad. Sci. 717: 1-15)

(Harman, 1998) (Harman D. Aging: phenomena and theories. *Ann NY Acad Sci* 854: 1-7, 1998)

(Harman, 2001) (Harman D. Aging: overview. *Ann NY Acad Sci* 928: 1–21, 2001)

(Harman, 2003) (Harman D. The free radical theory of aging. *Antioxid Redox Signal* 5: 557–561, 2003).

(Harman, 2009) (Harman, D. Origin and evolution of the free radial theory of aging: a brief personal history, 1954-2009. *Biogerontology* (2009) 10: 773-781)

(Hendin et al, 1999) (Hendin BN, Kolettis PN, Sharma RK, Thomas AJ, Jr., Agarwal A. Varicocele is associated with elevated spermatozoal reactive oxygen species production and diminished seminal plasma antioxidant capacity. *Journal of Urology.* 1999;161(6):1831–1834)

(Hietanen et al, 1994) (Hietanen E, Bartsch H, Bereziat JC, Camus AM, McClinton S, Eremin O, Davidson L, Boyle P. Diet and oxidative stress in breast, colon and prostate cancer patients: a case-control study. *Eur J Clin Nutr.* 1994;48: 575 -586)

(Holmes et al, 1992) (Holmes RP, Goodman HO, Shihabi ZK, Jarow JP. The taurine and hypotaurine content of human semen. J Androl. 1992;13:289–92)

(Howes, 2004) (Howes, R. M. © 2004. U.T.O.P.I.A. - Unified Theory of Oxygen Participation in Aerobiosis. Free Radical Publishing Co. Kentwood, LA)

(Howes, 2005) (Howes, R.M. © 2005. The Medical and Scientific Significance of Oxygen Free Radical Metabolism. Free Radical Publishing Co. Kentwood, LA)

(Howes, 2006, H2O2) (Howes, R.M. Hydrogen Peroxide Monograph 1: Scientific, Medical and Biochemical Overview & Monograph 2: Antioxidant Vitamins A, C, & E: Equivocal Scientific Studies, © 2006. Free Radical Publishing Co. Kentwood, LA)

(Howes, 2006, CVD) (Howes, R.M. Cardiovascular Disease and Oxygen Free Radical Mythology. © 2006. Free Radical Publishing Co. Kentwood, LA)

(Howes, 2006, Diabetes) (Howes, R.M. Diabetes and Oxygen Free Radical Sophistry. © 2006. Free Radical Publishing Co. Kentwood, LA)

(Howes, 2006, *Ann. N. Y. Acad. Sci.*) (Howes, R.M. The Free Radical Fantasy: A Panopoly of Paradoxes. *Ann. N. Y. Acad. Sci.* 2006;1067:22-26)

(Howes R.M. 2009, Am J Cosm Surg) (Howes, RM. Antioxidant Vitamins: A Review of Policy Statements and Recommendations. *The American Journal of Cosmetic Surgery.* 2009;26(2):63-78)

(Hsieh et al, 19980 (Hsieh, C. Y., Santell, R. C., Haslam, S. Z., Helferich, W. G., Estrogenic effects of genistein on the growth of estrogen receptor-positive human breast cancer (MCF-7) cells in vitro and in vivo. Cancer Res. 1998, 58, 3833–3838)

(Hughes et al, 1998) (Hughes CM, Lewis SE, McKelvey-Martin VJ, Thompson W. The effects of antioxidant supplementation during Percoll preparation on human sperm DNA integrity. Hum Reprod. 1998;13:1240–7)

(Irvine et al, 2000) (Irvine DS, Twigg JP, Gordon EL, Fulton N, Milne PA, Aitken RJ. DNA integrity in human spermatozoa: relationships with semen quality. J Androl. 2000;21:33–44)

(Iwanier, Zachara, 1995) (Iwanier K, Zachara BA. Selenium supplementation enhances the element concentration in blood and seminal fluid but does not change the spermatozoal quality characteristics in subfertile men. *J Androl.* 1995;16: 441 -447)

(Iwasaki, Gagnon, 1992) (Iwasaki A, Gagnon C. Formation of reactive oxygen species in spermatozoa of infertile patients. Fertil Steril. 1992;57:409–16)

(Jacob, 1990) (Jacob RA. Assessment of human vitamin C status. J Nutr. 1990;120(Suppl 11):1480–5)

(Jefferson et al, 2006) (Jefferson, W. N., Padilla-Banks, E., Newbold, R. R., Studies of the effects of neonatal exposure to genistein on the developing female reproductive system. J. AOAC Int. 2006, 89, 1189–1196)

(Jeulin et al, 1989) (Jeulin C, Soufir JC, Weber P, Laval-Martin D, Calvayrac R. Catalase activity in human spermatozoa and seminal plasma. Gamete Res. 1989;24:185–96)

(Jones et al, 2002) (Jones et al. Oxygen free radicals and the penis. Expert Opin Pharmacother. 2002 Jul;3(7):889-97)

(Jow et al, 1993) (Jow WW, Schlegel PN, Cichon Z, Phillips D, Goldstein M, Bardin CW. Identification and localization of copper-zinc superoxide dismutase gene expression in rat testicular development. J Androl. 1993;14:439–47)

(Ju et al, 2002) (Ju, Y. H., Doerge, D. R., Allred, K. F., Allred, C. D., Helferich, W. G., Dietary genistein negates the inhibitory effect of tamoxifen on growth of estrogen-dependent human breast cancer (MCF-7) cells implanted in athymic mice. Cancer Res. 2002, 62, 2474–2477)

(Ju et al, 2008) (Ju, Y. H., Doerge, D. R., Woodling, K. A., Hartman, J. A. et al., Dietary genistein negates the inhibitory effect of letrozole on the growth of aromatase-expressing estrogen-dependent human breast cancer cells (MCF-7Ca) in vivo. Carcinogenesis 2008, 29, 2162–2168)

(Kefer et al, 2009) (Kefer JC, Agarwal A, Sabanegh E. Role of antioxidants in the treatment of male infertility. *International Journal of Urology*. 2009;16(5):449–457)

(Keskes-Ammar et al, 2003) (Keskes-Ammar L, Feki-Chakroun N, Rebai T, Sahnoun Z, Ghozzi H, Hammami S, Zghal K, Fki H, Damak J, Bahloul A. Sperm oxidative stress and the effect of an oral vitamin E and selenium supplement on semen quality in infertile men. *Arch Androl.* 2003; 49: 83 -94)

(Kessopoulou et al, 1995) (Kessopoulou E, Powers HJ, Sharma KK, Pearson MJ, Russell JM, Cooke ID, Barratt CL. A double-blind randomized placebo cross-over controlled trial using the antioxidant vitamin E to treat reactive oxygen species associated male infertility. *Fertil Steril.* 1995; 64: 825 -831)

(Kim et al, 1993) (Kim N, Vardi Y, Padma-Nathan H, Daley J, Goldstein I, Saenz de Tejada I. Oxygen tension regulates the nitric oxide pathway. Physiological role in penile erection. *J Clin Invest* 91: 437–442, 1993)

(Kim et al, 1996) (Kim NN, Kim JJ, Hypolite J, García-Díaz JF, Broderick GA, Tornheim K, Daley JT, Levin R, Saenz de Tejada I. Altered contractility of rabbit penile corpus cavernosum smooth muscle by hypoxia. *J Urol* 155: 772–778, 1996)

(Kim et al, 2008) (Kim, Y. M., Yang, S., Xu, W., Li, S., Yang, X., Continuous in vitro exposure to low-dose genistein induces genomic instability in breast epithelial cells. Cancer Genet. Cytogenet. 2008, 186, 78–84)

(Kim et al, 2009) (Kim, D. J., Seok, S. H., Baek, M. W., Lee, H. Y. et al., Developmental toxicity and brain aromatase induction by high genistein concentrations in zebrafish embryos. Toxicol. Mech. Methods 2009, 19, 251–256)

(Kodama et al, 1996) (Kodama H, Kuribayashi Y, Gagnon C. Effect of sperm lipid peroxidation on fertilization. *Journal of Andrology*. 1996;17(2):151–157)

(Kodama et al, 1997) (Kodama H, Yamaguchi R, Fukuda J, Kasai H, Tanaka T. Increased oxidative deoxyribonucleic acid damage in the spermatozoa of infertile male patients. Fertil Steril. 1997;68:519–24)

(Kothari et al, 2010) (Kothari S, Thompson A, Agarwal A, du Plessis SS. Free radicals: their beneficial and detrimental effects on sperm function. Indian J Exp Biol. 2010 May;48(5):425-35)

(Kuhn et al., 1999) (Kuhn H, Thiele BJ. The diversity of the lipoxygenase family. Many sequence data but little information on biological significance. *FEBS Lett.* 1999;449:7–11)

(Kulling et al, 1999) (Kulling, S. E., Rosenberg, B., Jacobs, E., Metzler, M., The phytoestrogens coumoestrol and genistein induce structural chromosomal aberrations in cultured human peripheral blood lymphocytes. Arch. Toxicol. 1999, 73, 50–54)

(Kumar, Mahmood, 2001) (Kumar H, Mahmood S. The use of fast acting antioxidants for the reduction of cow placental retention and subsequent endometritis. *Indian Journal of Animal Sciences.* 2001;71(7):650–653)

(Lee et al, 2004) (Duk-Hee Lee, Aaron R Folsom, Lisa Harnack, Barry Halliwell and David R Jacobs, Jr. Does supplemental vitamin C increase cardiovascular disease risk in women with diabetes? American Journal of Clinical Nutrition, Vol. 80, No. 5, 1194-1200, November 2004)

(Lee et al., 1999) (Lee YJ, Shacter E. Oxidative stress inhibits apoptosis in human lymphoma cells. *J Biol Chem.* 1999;274:19792–19798)

(Lenzi et al, 1993) (Lenzi A, Culasso F, Gandini L, Lombardo F, Dondero F. Placebo-controlled, double-blind, cross-over trial of glutathione therapy in male infertility. *Hum Reprod.* 1993; 8: 1657 -1662)

(Lewin, Lavon, 1997) (Lewin A, Lavon H. The effect of coenzyme Q10 on sperm motility and function. *Mol Aspects Med.* 1997; 18(suppl): S213 -S219)

(Lewis et al, 1995) (Lewis SE, Boyle PM, McKinney KA, Young IS, Thompson W. Total antioxidant capacity of seminal plasma is different in fertile and infertile men. Fertil Steril. 1995;64:868–70)

(Lewis et al, 1997) (Lewis SE, Sterling ES, Young IS, Thompson W. Comparison of individual antioxidants of sperm and seminal plasma in fertile and infertile men. *Fertil Steril.* 1997; 67: 142 -147)

(Limer et al, 2006) (Limer, J. L., Parkes, A. T., Speirs, V., Differential response to phytoestrogens in endocrine sensitive and resistant breast cancer cells in vitro. Int. J. Cancer 2006, 119, 515–521)

(Liu et al, 2005) (Liu, B., Edgerton, S., Yang, X., Kim, A. et al., Low-dose dietary phytoestrogen abrogates tamoxifen-associated mammary tumor prevention. Cancer Res. 2005, 65, 879–886)

(Lombardo et al, 2011) (Lombardo et al. The role of antioxidant therapy in the treatment of male infertility: an overview. Asian J Androl. 2011 Jun 20. doi: 10.1038/aja.2010.183)

(Lopes et al, 1998) (Lopes S, Jurisicova A, Sun JG, Casper RF. Reactive oxygen species: potential cause for DNA fragmentation in human spermatozoa. Hum Reprod. 1998;13:896–900)

(Lopes et al, 2010) (Lopes AS, Lane M, Thompson JG. Oxygen consumption and ROS production are increased at the time of fertilization and cell cleavage in bovine zygotes. Hum Reprod. 2010 Nov;25(11):2762-73)

(Luo et al, 2006) (Luo Q, et al, Lycium barbarum polysaccharides: Protective effects against heat-induced damage of rat testes and H2O2-induced DNA damage in mouse testicular cells and beneficial effect on sexual behavior and reproductive function of hemicastrated rats. Life Sci. 2006 Jul 10;79(7):613-21)

(Manna, Samanta, 2003) (Manna I, Jana K, Samanta PK. Effect of intensive exercise-induced testicular gametogenic and steroidogenic disorders in mature male Wistar strain rats: A correlative approach to oxidative stress. *Acta Physiol Scand.* 2003;178:33–40)

(McMichael-Phillips et al, 1998) (McMichael-Phillips, D. F., Harding, C., Morton, M., Roberts, S. A. et al., Effects of soy-protein supplementation on epithelial proliferation in the histologically normal human breast. Am. J Clin. Nutr. 1998, 68, 1431S–1435S)

(Markovits et al, 1989) (Markovits, J., Linassier, C., Fosse, P., Couprie, J. et al., Inhibitory effects of the tyrosine kinase inhibitor genistein on mammalian DNA topoisomerase II. Cancer Res. 1989, 49, 5111–5117)

(Martin-Du Pan, Sakkas, 1998) (Martin-Du Pan RC, Sakkas D. Is antioxidant therapy a promising strategy to improve human reproduction? Are antioxidants useful in the treatment of male infertility? *Hum Reprod.* 1998; 13: 2984-2985)

(Meeker et al, 2010) (Meeker JD, et al. Semen quality and sperm DNA damage in relation to urinary bisphenol A among men from an infertility clinic. Reprod Toxicol. 2010 Dec;30(4):532-9)

(Meldrum et al, 2010) (Meldrum DR, Gambone JC, Morris MA, Ignarro LJ. A multifaceted approach to maximize erectile function and vascular health. Fertil Steril. 2010 Dec;94(7):2514-20)

(Menezo et al, 2007) (Menezo YJ, Hazout A, Panteix G, Robert F, Rollet J, Cohen-Bacrie P, et al. Antioxidants to reduce sperm DNA fragmentation: an unexpected adverse effect. Reprod Biomed Online. 2007;14:418–21)

(Michael et al, 2006) (Michael McClain, R., Wolz, E., Davidovich, A., Bausch, J., Genetic toxicity studies with genistein. Food Chem. Toxicol. 2006, 44, 42–55)

(Michel, Feron, 1997) (Michel T, Feron O. Nitric oxide synthases: which, where, how, and why?. *J Clin Invest.* Nov 1 1997;100(9):2146-52)

(Michelakis et al, 2002) (Michelakis ED, Hampl V, Nsair A, Wu X, Harry G, Haromy A, Gurtu R, Archer SL. Diversity in mitochondrial function explains differences in vascular oxygen sensing. *Circ Res* 90: 1307–1315, 2002)

(Miller et al, 1993) (Miller JK, Brzezinska-Slebodzinska E, Madsen FC. Oxidative stress, antioxidants, and animal function. *Journal of Dairy Science.* 1993;76(9):2812–2823)

(Miller et al., 2006) (Miller AA, Drummond GR, Sobey CG. Reactive oxygen species in the cerebral circulation: are they all bad? *Antioxid Redox Signal.* 2006;8:1113–1120)

(Miller et al, 2009) (Miller AA, Drummond GR, De Silva TM, Mast AE, Hickey H, Williams JP, Broughton BR, Sobey CG. NADPH oxidase activity is higher in cerebral versus systemic arteries of four animal species: role of Nox2. *Am J Physiol Heart Circ Physiol* 296: H220–H225, 2009)

(Mishra, Acharya, 2004) (Mishra M, Acharya UR. Protective action of vitamins on the spermatogenesis in lead treated Swiss mice. 2004. J. Trace Elem. Med. Biol. 18(2):173-8)

(Moilanen, Hovatta, 1995) (Moilanen J, Hovatta O. Excretion of alpha-tocopherol into human seminal plasma after oral administration. *Andrologia.* 1995; 27: 133 -136)

(Morton, 1995) (Morton RS. Sexual attitudes, preferences and infections in ancient Egypt. Genitourin Med 1995;71:180-6)

(Muratori et al, 2000) (Muratori M, Piomboni P, Baldi E, Filimberti E, Pecchioli P, Moretti E, et al. Functional and ultrastructural features of DNA-fragmented human sperm. J Androl. 2000;21:903–12)

(Mursu et al, 2011) (Mursu J, Robien K, Harnack LJ, Park K, Jacobs DR Jr. Dietary supplements and mortality rate in older women: the Iowa Women's Health Study. Arch Intern Med. 2011;171:1625-1633)

(Navaroa et al, 2005) (Navarová J, Ujházy E, Dubovický M, Mach M. Phenytoin induced oxidative stress in pre- and postnatal rat development - effect of vitamin E on selective biochemical variables. Biomed Pap Med Fac Univ Palacky Olomouc Czech Repub. 2005 Dec;149(2):325-8)

(Nunn, 1996) (Nunn JF. Ancient Egyptian medicine. British Museum Press, 1996)

(Ochendorf, 1999) (Ochendorf F.R. Infections in the male genital tract and reactive oxygen species. Human Reproduction Update 1999, Vol. 5, N0.5 p. 399-420)

(Ogawa et al., 2003) (Ogawa Y, Kobayashi T, Nishioka A, Kariya S, Hamasato S, Seguchi H, Yoshida S. Radiation-induced oxidative DNA damage, 8-oxoguanine, in human peripheral T cells. *Int J Mol Med.* 2003;11:27–32)

(Pakrashi et al, 1991) (Pakrashi A, Ray H, Pal BC, Mahato SB. Sperm immobilizing effect of triterpene saponins from Acacia auriculiformis. Contraception 1991;43:475-83)

(Pasqualotto et al, 2000) (Pasqualotto FF, Sharma RK, Potts JM, Nelson DR, Thomas AJ, Jr., Agarwal A. Seminal oxidative stress in patients with chronic prostatitis. *Urology.* 2000;55(6):881–885)

(Piomboni et al, 2008) (Piomboni P, Gambera L, Serafini F, Campanella G, Morgante G, De Leo V. Sperm quality improvement after natural antioxidant treatment of asthenoteratospermic men with leukocytospermia. Asian J Androl. 2008;10:201–6)

(Podmore et al, 1998) (Podmore ID, Griffiths HR, Herbert KE, Mistry N, Mistry P, Lunec J. Vitamin C exhibits pro-oxidant properties. *Nature.* 1998;392:559)

(Pool-Zobel et al, 2000) (Pool-Zobel, B. L., Adlercreutz, H., Glei, M., Liegibel, U. M. et al., Isoflavonoids and lignans have different potentials to modulate oxidative genetic damage in human colon cells. Carcinogenesis 2000, 21, 1247–1252)

(Potts et al, 2000) (Potts RJ, Notarianni LJ, Jefferies TM. Seminal plasma reduces exogenous oxidative damage to human sperm, determined by the measurement of DNA strand breaks and lipid peroxidation. Mutat Res. 2000;447:249–56)

(Potts, Pasaqualotto, 2003) (Potts JM, Pasqualotto FF. Seminal oxidative stress in patients with chronic prostatitis. 2003. Andrologia 35:304-308)

(Potts et al, 2004) (Potts RJ, Notarianni LJ, Jefferies TM. Seminal plasma reduces exogenous oxidative damage to human sperm, determined by the measurement of DNA strand breaks and lipid peroxidation. Mutat Res. 2000;447:249–56)

(Prieto et al, 2010) (Prieto D et al. Hypoxic relaxation of penile arteries: involvement of endothelial nitric oxide and modulation by reactive oxygen species. Am J Physiol Heart Circ Physiol. 2010 Sep;299(3):H915-24)

(Ramalho-Santos et al, 2009) (Ramalho-Santos et al, Mitochondrial functionality in reproduction: from gonads and gametes to embryos and embryonic stem cells. Hum. Reprod. Update (2009)15(5):553-572)

(Ramsey et al, 2001) (Ramsey KH, et al. Role for Inducible Nitric Oxide Synthase in Protection from Chronic *Chlamydia trachomatis* Urogenital Disease in Mice and Its Regulation by Oxygen Free Radicals. Infect Immun. 2001 December; 69(12): 7374–7379)

(Reeves, 1992) (Reeves C. Egyptian medicine. Shire Publications, 1992)

(Reiter et al, 2008) (Reiter et al. Melatonin combats molecular terrorism at the mitochondrial level. Interdiscip Toxicol 2008 Sep;1(2):137-49)

(Rhee et al., 2003) (Rhee SG, Chang TS, Bae YS, Lee SR, Kang SW. Cellular regulation by hydrogen peroxide. *J Am Soc Nephrol.* 2003;14:S211–S215)

(Rhee, 2006) (Rhee SG. H_2O_2, a necessary evil for cell signaling. *Science.* 2006;312(5782):1882–1883)

(Rolf et al, 1999) (Rolf C, Cooper TG, Yeung CH, Nieschlag E. Antioxidant treatment of patients with asthenozoospermia or moderate oligoasthenozoospermia with high-dose vitamin C and vitamin E: a randomized, placebo-controlled, double-blind study. *Hum Reprod.* 1999; 14: 1028 -1033)

(Romm, 1999) (Romm JS. Herodotus. 1st ed. Yale University Press, 1999)

(Ruder et al, 2008) (Ruder EH, et al. Oxidative stress and antioxidants: exposure and impact on female fertility. Human Reproduction Update, Vol. 14, No. 4 pp. 345-357, 2008)

(Russo et al, 2006) (Russo A, Troncoso N, Sanchez F, Garbarino JA, Vanella A. Propolis protects human spermatozoa from DNA damage caused by benzo[a] pyrene and exogenous reactive oxygen species. Life Sci. 2006;78:1401–6)

(Ryle, Thompson, 1984) (Ryle PR, Thomson AD. Nutrition and vitamins in alcoholism. Contemp Issues Clin Biochem. 1984;1:188–224).

(Sadovosky et al, 2008) (Sadovsky R, et al. Patient use of dietary supplements: a clinician's perspective. Curr Med Res Opin. 2008 Apr;24(4):1209-16)

(Said et al, 2005) (Said TM, Agarwal A, Sharma RK, Thomas AJ Jr, Sikka SC. Impact of sperm morphology on DNA damage caused by oxidative stress induced by beta-nicotinamide adenine dinucleotide phosphate. Fertil Steril. 2005;83:95–103)

(Saito et al., 2006) (Saito Y, Nishio K, Ogawa Y, Kimata J, Kinumi T, Yoshida Y, Noguchi N, Niki E. Turning point in apoptosis/necrosis induced by hydrogen peroxide. *Free Radic Res.* 2006;40:619–630)

(Sakkas et al, 1998) (Sakkas D, Urner F, Bizzaro D, et al. Sperm nuclear DNA damage and altered chromatin structure: effect on fertilization and embryo development. *Human Reproduction.* 1998;13(supplement 4):11–19)

(Sakkas et al, 2003) (Sakkas D, Seli E, Bizzaro D, Tarozzi N, Manicardi GC. Abnormal spermatozoa in the ejaculate: abortive apoptosis and faulty nuclear remodelling during spermatogenesis. Reprod Biomed Online. 2003;7:428–32)

(Saleh et al, 2002) (Saleh RA, Agarwal A, Kandirali E, et al. Leukocytospermia is associated with increased reactive oxygen species production by human spermatozoa. *Fertility and Sterility.* 2002;78(6):1215–1224)

(Saleh et al, 2003) (Saleh RA, Agarwal A, Sharma RK, Said TM, Sikka SC, Thomas AJ Jr. Evaluation of nuclear DNA damage in spermatozoa from infertile men with varicocele. Fertil Steril. 2003;80:1431–6)

(Sanocka et al, 1996) (Sanocka D, Miesel R, Jedrzejczak P, Kurpisz MK. Oxidative stress and male infertility. J Androl. 1996;17:449–54)

(Sanocka et al, 1997) (Sanocka D, Miesel R, Jedrzejczak P, Chelmonska-Soyta AC, Kurpisz M. Effect of reactive oxygen species and the activity of antioxidant systems on human semen; association with male infertility. Int J Androl. 1997;20:255–64)

(Sanocka, Kurpisz, 2004) (Sanocka D, Kurpisz M. Reactive oxygen species and sperm cells. *Reproductive Biology and Endocrinology.* 2004;2:12–26)

(Sassi-Messai et al, 2009) (Sassi-Messai, S., Gibert, Y., Bernard, L., Nishio, S. et al., The phytoestrogen genistein affects zebrafish development through two different pathways. PloS ONE 2009, 4, e4935)

(Sati et al, 2008) (Sati L, Ovari L, Bennett D, Simon SD, Demir R, Huszar G. Double probing of human spermatozoa for persistent histones, surplus cytoplasm, apoptosis and DNA fragmentation. Reprod Biomed Online. 2008;16:570–9)

(Sawyer et al, 2003) (Sawyer DE, Mercer BG, Wiklendt AM, Aitken RJ. Quantitative analysis of gene-specific DNA damage in human spermatozoa. Mutat Res. 2003;529:21–34)

(Semple et al, 1984) (Semple PD et al. Sex hormone suppression and sexual impotence in hypoxic pulmonary fibrosis. Thorax. 1984 Jan;39(1):46-51)

(Shalika et al, 1996) (Shalika S, Dugan K, Smith RD, Padilla SL. The effect of positive semen bacterial and Ureaplasma cultures on in-vitro fertilization success. *Human Reproduction.* 1996;11(12):2789–2792)

(Sharma, Agarwal, 1996) (Sharma RK, Agarwal A. Role of reactive oxygen species in male infertility. 1996. Urology 48(6):835-850)

(Sharma et al, 2001) (Sharma RK, Pasqualotto FF, Nelson DR, Thomas AJ, Jr., Agarwal A. Relationship between seminal white blood cell counts and oxidative stress in men treated at an infertility clinic. *Journal of Andrology.* 2001;22(4):575–583)

(Sharma, Agarwal, 1996) (Sharma RK, Agarwal A. Role of reactive oxygen species in male infertility. *Urology.* 1996;48(6):835–850)

(Shen et al, 1999) (Shen HM, Chia SE, Ong CN. Evaluation of oxidative DNA damage in human sperm and its association with male infertility. J Androl. 1999;20:718–23)

(Sherrill et al, 2010) (Sherrill, J. D., Sparks, M., Dennis, J., Mansour, M. et al., Developmental exposures of male rats to soy isoflavones impact leydig cell differentiation. Biol. Reprod. 2010, 83, 488–501)

(Shokeir, Hussein, 2004) (Shokeir AA, Hussein MI. Sexual life in Pharaonic Egypt: towards a urological view. Int J Impot Res 2004;16:385-8)

(Sierens et al, 2002) (Sierens J, Hartley JA, Campbell MJ, Leathem AJ, Woodside JV. In vitro isoflavone supplementation reduces hydrogen peroxide-induced DNA damage in sperm. Teratog Carcinog Mutagen. 2002;22:227–34)

(Sigman et al, 2009) (Sigman M, Baazeem A, Zini A. Semen analysis and sperm function assays: what do they mean? Semin Reprod Med. 2009 Mar;27(2):115-23)

(Sikka, 1996) (Sikka SC. Oxidative stress and role of antioxidants in normal and abnormal sperm function. *Frontiers in Bioscience.* 1996;1:e78–e86)

(Sikka, 2001) (Sikka SC. Relative impact of oxidative stress on male reproductive function. *Current Medicinal Chemistry.* 2001;8(7):851–862)

(Silver et al, 2005) (Silver EW, Eskenazi B, Evenson DP, Block G, Young S, Wyrobek AJ. Effect of antioxidant intake on sperm chromatin stability in healthy nonsmoking men. J Androl. 2005;26:550–6)

(Smith et al, 1996) (Smith R, Vantman D, Ponce J, Escobar J, Lissi E. Total antioxidant capacity of human seminal plasma. Hum Reprod. 1996;11:1655–60)

(Song et al, 2008) (Song GJ, Lewis V. Mitochondrial DNA integrity and copy number in sperm from infertile men. Fertil Steril. 2008;90:2238–44)

(Sonmez et al, 2005) (Sonmez M, Turk G, Yuce A. The effect of ascorbic acid supplementation on sperm quality, lipid peroxidation, and testosterone levels in male Wistar rats. 2005. Theriogenology. 63(7): 2063-72)

(Strzezek et al, 2004) (Strzezek J, Fraser L, Kuklinska M, Dziekonska A, Lecewicz M. Effects of dietary supplementation with polyunsaturated fatty acids and antioxidants on biochemical characteristics of boar semen. 2004. Repro. Biol. 4(3):271-87)

(Tarin et al, 1998) (Tarín JJ, Brines J, Cano A. Is antioxidant therapy a promising strategy to improve human reproduction? *Human Reproduction.* 1998;13(6):1415–1424)

(Taylor et al, 2009) (Taylor K, Roberts P, Sanders K, Burton P. Effect of antioxidant supplementation of cryopreservation medium on post-thaw integrity of human spermatozoa. Reprod Biomed Online. 2009;18:184–9)

(Taylor, Levy et al, 2009) (Taylor, C. K., Levy, R. M., Elliott, J. C., Burnett, B. P., The effect of genistein aglycone on cancer and cancer risk: a review of in vitro, preclinical, and clinical studies. Nutr. Rev. 2009, 67, 398–415)

(Toda et al, 2005) (Toda N, et al. Nitric oxide and penile erectile function. Pharmacol Ther. 2005 May;106(2):233-66)

(Tonks et al., 2005) (Tonks NK. 2005. Redox redux: revisiting PTPs and the control of cell signalling. *Cell.* 2005;121:667–670)

(Torres, Velando 2007) (Torres R, Velando A. Male reproductive senescence: the price of immune-induced oxidative damage on sexual attractiveness in the blue-footed booby. J Anim Ecol. 2007 Nov;76(6):1161-8)

(Tremellen et al, 2007) (Tremellen K, et al. A randomised control trial examining the effect of an antioxidant (Menevit) on pregnancy outcome during IVF-ICSI treatment. Aust N Z J Obstet Gynaecol. 2007 Jun;47(3):216-21)

(Twigg et al, 1998) (Twigg J, Fulton N, Gomez E, Irvine DS, Aitken RJ. Analysis of the impact of intracellular reactive oxygen species generation on the structural and functional integrity of human spermatozoa: lipid peroxidation, DNA fragmentation and effectiveness of antioxidants. Hum Reprod. 1998;13:1429–36)

(Valicenti et al, 2002) (Valicenti RK, Bissonette EA, Chen C, Theodorescu D. Longitudinal comparison of sexual function after 3-dimensional conformal radiation therapy or prostate brachytherapy. J Urol. Dec 2002;168(6):2499-504; discussion 2504)

(Valko et al, 2005) (Valko M, Morris H, Cronin MTD. Metals, toxicity and oxidative stress. Current Medicinal Chemistry. 2005;12(10):1161–1208)

(Van Heerebeek et al., 2002) (Van Heerebeek L, Meischl C, Stooker W, Meijer CJ, Niessen HW, Roos D. NADPH oxidase(s): new source(s) of reactive oxygen species in the vascular system? J Clin Pathol. 2002;55:561–568)

(Verit et at, 2006) (Verit FF, Verit A, Kocyigit A, Ciftci H, Celik H, Koksal M. No increase in sperm DNA damage and seminal oxidative stress in patients with idiopathic infertility. Arch Gynecol Obstet. 2006;274:339–44)

(Vernet et al, 2004) (Vernet P, Aitken RD, Drevet JR. Antioxidant strategies in the epididymis. 2004. Mol. Cell. Endocrin. 216:31-39).

(Wang et al, 1997) (Wang Y, Sharma RK, Agarwal A. Effect of cryopreservation and sperm concentration on lipid peroxidation in human semen. Urology. 1997;50(3):409–413)

(Wisniewski et al, 2003) (Wisniewski, A. B., Klein, S. L., Lakshmanan, Y., Gearhart, J. P., Exposure to genistein during gestation and lactation demasculinizes the reproductive system in rats. J. Urol. 2003, 169, 1582–1586)

(Wolin, 2009) (Wolin MS. Reactive oxygen species and the control of vascular function. Am J Physiol Heart Circ Physiol 296: H539–H549, 2009)

(Wong et al, 2004) (Wong, , JL, Creton R, Wessel GM. 2004. The oxidative burst at fertilization is dependent upon activation of the dual oxidase UdxI. Dev. Cwell. 7:801-814)

(Xu et al, 2003) (Xu DX, Shen HM, Zhu QX, Chua L, Wang QN, Chia SE, et al. The associations among semen quality, oxidative DNA damage in human spermatozoa and concentrations of cadmium, lead and selenium in seminal plasma. Mutat Res. 2003;534:155–63)

(Young et al, 2008) (Young SS, et al. The association of folate, zinc and antioxidant intake with sperm aneuploidy in healthy non-smoking men. Hum Reprod. 2008 May;23(5):1014-22)

(Yousef et al, 2003) (Yousef MI, Abdallah GA, Kamel KI. Effect of ascorbic acid and Vitamin E supplementation on semen quality and biochemical parameters of male rabbits. *Animal Reproduction Science.* 2003;76(1-2):99–111)

(Zini et al, 1993) (Zini A, de Lamirande E, Gagnon C. Reactive oxygen species in semen of infertile patients: levels of superoxide dismutase- and catalase-like activities in seminal plasma and spermatozoa. Int J Androl. 1993;16:183–8)

(Zini et al, 1996) (Zini A, Schlegel PN. Catalase mRNA expression in the male rat reproductive tract. J Androl. 1996;17:473–80)

(Zini, Schlegel, 1997) (Zini A, Schlegel PN. Identification and characterization of antioxidant enzyme mRNAs in the rat epididymis. Int J Androl. 1997;20:86–91)

(Zini et al, 1997) (Zini A, Schlegel PN. Expression of glutathione peroxidases in the adult male rat reproductive tract. Fertil Steril. 1997;68:689–95)

(Zini et al, 2005) (Zini A, Blumenfeld A, Libman J, Willis J. Beneficial effect of microsurgical varicocelectomy on human sperm DNA integrity. Hum Reprod. 2005;20:1018–21)

(Zini et al, 2009) (Zini A, San Gabriel M, Baazeem A. Antioxidants and sperm DMA damage: a clinical perspective. J. Assist Reprod Genet. 2009 Aug;26(8):427-32)

(Zini et al, 2009) (Zini A, San Gabriel M, Baazeem A. Antioxidants and sperm DMA damage: a clinical perspective. J. Assist Reprod Genet. 2009 Aug;26(8):427-32)

(Zini, Al-Hathal, 2011) (Zini A, Al-Hathal N. Antioxidant therapy in male infertility: fact or fiction? Asian J Androl. 2011 May;13(3):374-81)

(Zhang et al, 2011) (Zhang Q, et al. Dietary antioxidants improve arteriogenic erectile dysfunction. Int J Androl. 2011 Jun;34(3):225-35)

(Zribi et al, 2011) (Zribi N, et al, Sperm DNA fragmentation and oxidation are independent of malondialdheyde. Reprod Biol Endocrinol. 2011 Apr 14;9:47)